Perfectionism Detox Workbook

9 Practical Strategies to Alleviate Stress, Manage Anxiety, and Reclaim Your Time for What Really Matters

Dr. Stacey Bottone

Perfectionism Detox Workbook:

9 Practical Strategies to Alleviate Stress, Manage Anxiety, and Reclaim Your Time for What Really Matters

To Josh, my rock and greatest supporter. Your unwavering belief in me has been my strength through every challenge. Thank you for your love, patience, and encouragement.

Table of Contents

Introduction

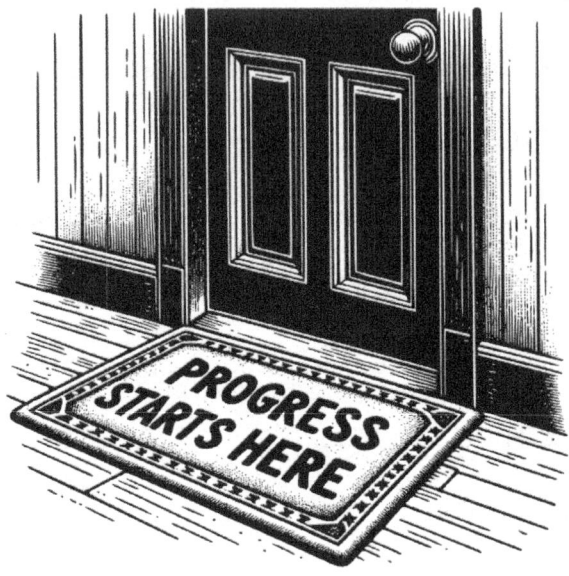

The alarm clock buzzes. Another day begins, and before you've even had your coffee, your mind races with everything you need to do. That endless to-do list looms overhead, and no matter how hard you try, it feels like there's always something left undone. You tell yourself, "I just need to work harder, stay more focused, or be better organized." But deep down, you wonder if even that will be enough. Sound familiar?

Welcome to the perfectionism trap—a cycle that leaves you constantly striving yet never fully satisfied. Perfectionism often wears a mask, disguising itself as a quest for excellence or ambition. But the truth is, it can rob you of joy, energy, and time—especially the time you'd rather spend on the people and things that truly matter.

1

I know this struggle firsthand. As someone who has battled the pressures of perfectionism in both my career and personal life, I've been there: the late nights obsessing over details, the fear of falling short, and the exhaustion of trying to meet impossible standards. It took time, but I found a way to step off the treadmill. This workbook is the culmination of years of research, self-discovery, and practical strategies I've developed to help others do the same.

This isn't about lowering your standards or giving up on your goals. It's about redefining success in a way that allows you to thrive—not just achieve. Through nine practical strategies, you'll learn to quiet the perfectionist voice in your head, manage stress, and reclaim your energy for what matters most.

Each chapter includes case studies, actionable steps, and over 150 total interactive exercises to help you apply the concepts to your own life. But don't feel pressured to complete every activity. This is your personal journey, and you can choose the exercises that resonate with you or fit into your schedule. The goal isn't to overwhelm you with tasks—it's to provide you with tools to make meaningful progress at your own pace.

Along the way, you'll reflect, experiment, and have the tools to make real changes. Most importantly, you'll practice self-compassion—a skill as critical as any strategy in this book.

This journey isn't about becoming perfect at overcoming perfectionism. It's about progress. So let's take that first step together and start rewriting the story. You don't have to do this perfectly—you just have to begin.

Understanding Your Perfectionism

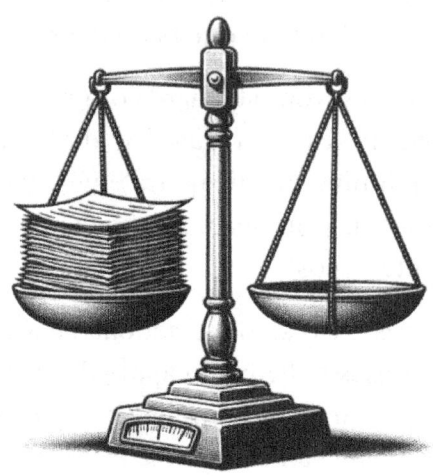

You're in a meeting, your heart racing as you mentally review every word of your presentation, convinced everyone is noticing flaws that only you can see. Later, you check off your tasks for the day, feeling a brief moment of satisfaction. But it's fleeting. Instead of celebrating your accomplishments, you focus on what you could have done better. Sound familiar? This is the exhausting cycle of perfectionism, and it's something many of us know all too well.

In this chapter, we'll uncover what drives perfectionism and how it manifests in our daily lives. By understanding its roots, you'll be better equipped to begin shifting your mindset and habits.

1.1 What Fuels Perfectionism?

Perfectionism isn't just about wanting to do things well—it's about a deeper, more intricate interplay of internal and external influences that shape our behaviors and beliefs. To truly address perfectionism, we need to understand where it comes from. By examining the roots of perfectionism, we can begin to identify patterns and develop healthier approaches to our goals.

Family and Upbringing

Perfectionism often begins in childhood, influenced by family dynamics and early experiences. Were you praised for accomplishments but criticized for falling short? For many, childhood experiences create the blueprint for how they perceive success and failure. Parents or caregivers may have unintentionally reinforced perfectionist tendencies by emphasizing outcomes rather than effort. Comments like "You're so smart" or "Why didn't you get an A+?" might have seemed harmless but can send the message that your value is tied to your achievements.

In households with high expectations, children may feel immense pressure to excel academically, athletically, or socially. The fear of disappointing loved ones can make failure feel catastrophic. Alternatively, growing up in an unpredictable or critical environment might lead some to seek control through perfectionism. If mistakes were met with harsh consequences, striving for flawlessness can feel like a way to avoid criticism or maintain a sense of safety.

Even siblings can shape our perfectionist tendencies. Comparisons within families—whether direct ("Why can't you be more like your brother?") or implied—can instill the belief that you need to be the best to stand out or gain approval.

Cultural Expectations and Societal Pressures

Beyond the family, society plays a significant role in fostering perfectionism. In many cultures, excellence is celebrated, and mediocrity is frowned upon. The idea that you must "be the best" permeates every aspect of life, from academics to career achievements to personal milestones. This can create a relentless cycle of striving without ever feeling satisfied.

Social media has amplified these pressures tenfold. Platforms like Instagram, TikTok, and LinkedIn provide a constant stream of curated perfection—flawless bodies, enviable lifestyles, and unblemished professional achievements. What we often forget is that these glimpses are heavily edited and far from reality. However, the endless comparison can make you feel inadequate, as if everyone else is achieving more with less effort.

Workplace cultures can also reinforce perfectionism. Companies that reward overwork, celebrate "hustle culture," or prioritize results over well-being can create environments where employees feel they must be perfect to succeed. In such settings, even minor mistakes can feel like personal failures.

Internal Drives and Personality Traits

Some individuals are naturally predisposed to perfectionism due to their personality traits. Traits like conscientiousness, high sensitivity, and a strong sense of responsibility can make someone more likely to develop perfectionist tendencies. While these characteristics often lead to success, they can also become double-edged swords when perfectionism takes hold.

For example, if you're naturally detail-oriented, you may struggle to let go of projects, endlessly revising and refining to ensure they're "just right." If you have a strong desire to please others, you might prioritize their expectations over your well-being. These internal drives can create a cycle where nothing ever feels good enough.

The Role of Conditional Approval

A recurring theme in perfectionism is the experience of conditional approval—feeling loved or valued only when you succeed. This can manifest in subtle ways, such as receiving praise only for achievements or being overlooked unless you excel. Over time, you might internalize the belief that your worth is tied to your performance, making the fear of failure even more intense.

Activity: Reflect on Your Roots

Understanding where your perfectionism comes from is a vital step toward managing it. Take some time to reflect on the following questions in your journal or notebook. Be honest and detailed in your responses:

1. **What messages about success and failure did you hear growing up?**
   Write down specific phrases or moments that stand out. For example, did your parents emphasize winning above all else? Did teachers praise your efforts or only your results?

2. **How do these messages influence your current behaviors?**
   Consider how your childhood experiences shape the way you approach your goals. Do you still feel the need to earn approval through achievements?

3. **What areas of your life feel the most pressure-packed?**
   Identify where you feel the strongest pull to be perfect—whether it's at work, in relationships, or in personal hobbies. Why do you think these areas carry so much weight?

4. **Who do you compare yourself to, and why?**
   Think about the people or images you often measure yourself against. Are they realistic benchmarks, or are they part of a perfectionist narrative?

This reflection exercise will help you uncover the hidden influences driving your perfectionism and allow you to start challenging them.

A Practical Example: Meet Sarah

Sarah, a 34-year-old marketing professional, always felt pressure to excel. Growing up, her parents celebrated her report cards and athletic achievements but rarely acknowledged her efforts when she fell short.

As an adult, Sarah finds herself obsessing over every detail in her work projects, fearing that one mistake could undermine her entire career.

When Sarah began reflecting on her perfectionism, she realized that much of it stemmed from her upbringing. Her parents' emphasis on results made her equate success with worthiness. She also recognized that her workplace culture, which rewarded perfectionism, reinforced these tendencies.

By acknowledging these influences, Sarah began to reframe her thinking. She focused on the value of her contributions rather than the need to avoid mistakes. Gradually, she found it easier to let go of her perfectionist habits, leading to less stress and more satisfaction in her work.

Building Awareness and Compassion

The key to addressing perfectionism is not to eliminate your drive for excellence but to understand its origins and impact. By recognizing the influences that shaped your perfectionism—family, society, internal drives—you can begin to separate healthy ambition from harmful expectations.

As you move forward, remember that perfectionism is not an unchangeable part of who you are. It's a learned behavior that can be unlearned with time, effort, and self-compassion. Each step you take toward understanding your perfectionism brings you closer to living a life that's guided by progress, not perfection.

1.2 The Many Faces of Perfectionism

Perfectionism isn't a one-size-fits-all experience. It manifests in distinct forms, each with unique characteristics and challenges. Understanding these types can help you identify how perfectionism affects your life.

Self-Oriented Perfectionism

If you constantly push yourself to excel and feel deeply dissatisfied with anything less than perfect, you're likely grappling with self-oriented perfectionism. This type often involves setting unrealistically high expectations for yourself and struggling with self-criticism when you don't meet them. While striving for personal growth is healthy, self-oriented perfectionism can lead to chronic dissatisfaction, as you feel like nothing is ever enough.

Example:

Imagine spending hours perfecting a report for work. Even after receiving praise from your boss, you fixate on the minor details you could have improved. This relentless self-scrutiny undermines your sense of accomplishment.

Socially Prescribed Perfectionism

Do you worry about what others think? Socially prescribed perfectionism stems from the belief that those around you demand perfection. This can create a paralyzing fear of failure, as you feel the weight of others' expectations bearing down on you.

Example:

You might feel compelled to host the perfect dinner party, fearing judgment from friends if the food isn't flawless or the house isn't spotless. The pressure to impress others can overshadow the joy of the occasion.

Other-Oriented Perfectionism

This type focuses on holding others to high standards. You might find yourself frustrated when colleagues don't meet your expectations or when friends don't share your meticulous attention to detail. While this can strain relationships, it often originates from a desire for order or excellence rather than malice.

Example:

A team project at work might leave you feeling exasperated if others don't meet your level of precision. This frustration can lead to micromanagement or conflict, affecting both the outcome and your relationships.

Interactive Activity: Mapping Your Perfectionism

To gain clarity on how perfectionism shows up in your life, create a chart with the following headings:

Type of Perfectionism	How It Shows Up in My Life	How it Impacts Me
Self-Oriented	I spend hours redoing tasks that are already good enough.	I feel exhausted and frustrated.
Socially Prescribed	I worry about being judged for small mistakes.	It makes me anxious and stressed.
Other-Oriented	I get irritated when others don't meet my standards.	It strains my relationships.

Filling out this chart with specific examples can help you better understand how perfectionism manifests and affects your well-being.

Expanding Understanding Through Reflection

Understanding these different types of perfectionism allows you to recognize how they interact and overlap. You might find that you identify with more than one type, depending on the context. For example, you may hold yourself to high standards at work (self-oriented) while also feeling pressure to meet others' expectations in social settings (socially prescribed).

This deeper understanding equips you to take the next steps in addressing perfectionism, whether it's learning to set realistic goals, challenging negative thought patterns, or building healthier relationships.

1.3 How Perfectionism Affects Your Life

Perfectionism is more than a mindset—it's a way of life that can permeate every area of your existence, shaping your emotions, decisions, and relationships. While striving for high standards can sometimes lead to positive outcomes, the relentless pursuit of flawlessness often comes with significant costs.

The Emotional Toll

Living under the constant pressure to be perfect creates a heightened state of stress. You may find yourself replaying past mistakes, agonizing over what you should have done differently, or worrying about how you'll avoid future errors. This mental strain can manifest as:

- **Anxiety:** The fear of failure or criticism can make even routine tasks feel overwhelming, as if every action carries immense weight.

- **Depression:** When you fall short of your own expectations, you may spiral into feelings of disappointment or self-blame, eroding your sense of self-worth.

- **Emotional Exhaustion:** Constantly striving to meet impossible standards drains your energy, leaving you feeling depleted and unable to fully enjoy your achievements.

Example:

Imagine preparing a dinner party for friends. Instead of enjoying the process of cooking and connecting, you obsess over every detail—the placement of utensils, the exact doneness of the roast, the perfection of the dessert. Even when your friends compliment the meal, you fixate on the imperfections, robbing yourself of the joy of the evening.

Activity: Recognizing Emotional Patterns

In your journal, write about a recent situation where perfectionism took an emotional toll. Consider the following prompts:

- What were you striving to achieve?

- How did your emotions shift throughout the process?

- What impact did your perfectionism have on your overall experience?

Procrastination and Paralysis

It's ironic that perfectionism, which pushes you to achieve, often leads to procrastination. The fear of not doing something "perfectly" can make starting a task feel daunting. You might delay until the last possible moment, creating a cycle of stress as the deadline looms. This avoidance doesn't just affect productivity—it amplifies feelings of failure and inadequacy.

- **Paralysis Before Starting:** The overwhelming need to get everything right can make a blank page or an untouched project feel insurmountable.

- **Last-Minute Scramble:** Putting tasks off often results in a frantic rush to finish, leaving little room for the perfection you initially sought.

- **Missed Opportunities:** Fear of imperfection can lead to avoiding risks altogether, stalling personal or professional growth.

Example:

Consider a student who delays starting an essay because they want it to be flawless. As the deadline nears, the pressure mounts, and they hastily complete the assignment, feeling unsatisfied with the result.

This cycle reinforces the belief that they can never meet their own high standards.

Interactive Exercise: Breaking the Cycle

1. Identify a task you've been avoiding.

2. Break it into small, manageable steps.

3. Commit to completing the first step today, focusing on progress rather than perfection.

4. Reflect on how it feels to make even a small amount of progress.

Struggles in Relationships

Perfectionism doesn't exist in a vacuum—it inevitably affects your interactions with others. Whether you impose high standards on loved ones or withdraw out of fear of judgment, perfectionism can create barriers in your relationships.

- **High Expectations:** You might unintentionally hold others to the same impossible standards you set for yourself. This can lead to frustration when they don't meet your expectations and strain your connections.

- **Fear of Vulnerability:** The need to appear perfect can make you hesitant to open up, creating distance between you and the people who care about you.

- **Isolation:** If you're overly critical of yourself or others, you may avoid social situations altogether, fearing judgment or rejection.

Example:

A parent who expects their child to excel in academics and extracurriculars might unintentionally place undue pressure on them. While the intention may be to encourage success, the child may feel inadequate or unloved when they fall short, straining the parent-child bond.

Activity: Relationship Reflection

Think about how perfectionism influences your relationships. Write down:

- An example of a time when your perfectionism created tension with someone close to you.

- How that situation could have been different if perfectionism hadn't been a factor.

- One step you can take to foster healthier, more open relationships moving forward.

Missed Opportunities for Growth

Perfectionism often disguises itself as a commitment to excellence, but it can also block your ability to take risks and grow. The fear of failure can prevent you from trying new things, exploring opportunities, or learning from mistakes. This stifling effect can hinder both personal and professional development.

Example:

Imagine turning down a chance to lead a project at work because you're afraid you won't do it perfectly. While this might feel like a safe choice in the moment, it could limit your career advancement and leave you wondering what might have been.

Interactive Activity: Redefining Success

Take a moment to redefine what success looks like for you. In your journal, answer these questions:

- What does progress look like, even if it's not perfect?

- How can mistakes or setbacks help you grow?

- What is one small risk you could take this week to step outside your comfort zone?

Reflection Exercise: Your Perfectionist Impact

To gain a clearer understanding of how perfectionism affects your life, spend time reflecting on these prompts:

1. **Mental Health:**

   o How has perfectionism influenced your stress, anxiety, or self-esteem?

   o Have you ever avoided seeking help because you didn't want to appear weak or flawed?

2. **Relationships:**

   o Are there times when your perfectionism created tension with loved ones or coworkers?

   o How do you think letting go of perfectionism could improve your relationships?

3. **Productivity:**

   o What tasks have you procrastinated on because of the fear of doing them imperfectly?

   o How has this procrastination affected your performance or sense of accomplishment?

Use your reflections as a starting point for identifying areas where you'd like to make changes. By recognizing the specific ways perfectionism impacts your life, you can begin to address its hold on you.

Expanding Your Understanding

As you consider the effects of perfectionism, it's important to remember that these patterns aren't fixed. While perfectionism may currently shape your emotions, decisions, and relationships, it doesn't have to define your future. With greater self-awareness and the tools provided in this workbook, you can start to shift these patterns and create a life that values progress over perfection. Each step you take is a step toward greater freedom and fulfillment.

1.4 Breaking the Perfectionism-Avoidance Cycle

Perfectionism and avoidance often go hand in hand. The fear of falling short can paralyze you, leading to procrastination or even abandonment of tasks. Breaking this cycle requires deliberate effort to shift your mindset, confront fears, and develop healthier habits.

Understanding the Avoidance Trap

Avoidance may feel like a temporary escape, but it creates a vicious cycle. The more you delay starting or finishing a task, the more overwhelming it becomes. This procrastination often results in last-minute scrambles, heightened anxiety, and less-than-satisfying outcomes. Over time, avoidance reinforces the belief that you're not capable, fueling the very perfectionism you're trying to escape.

Example:

Consider someone who avoids writing a report for work, fearing it won't meet their high standards. As the deadline approaches, they rush to complete it, feeling stressed and dissatisfied with the final product. This reinforces their belief that they're not good enough, perpetuating the cycle.

Reflection Exercise:

Think about a recent time you procrastinated on a task due to perfectionism. Ask yourself:

- What were you afraid of?
- How did avoidance impact the outcome?
- What could you have done differently?

Jot down your reflections in a journal to start identifying patterns in your avoidance behavior.

Reframing Your Thoughts

Your inner dialogue plays a significant role in perpetuating perfectionism. The critical voice in your head often magnifies flaws and minimizes successes. Reframing these thoughts is a powerful tool for breaking the cycle.

- **Identify Your Inner Critic:** Pay attention to the negative thoughts that surface when you're working on a task. Common themes include fear of failure, worry about others' opinions, or feelings of inadequacy.

- **Challenge and Reframe:** Once you've identified a negative thought, counter it with a more balanced perspective.

Examples of Thought Reframing:

- **Inner Critic:** "If I don't get this exactly right, I'll disappoint everyone."
  Reframe: "Doing my best is enough, and most people will appreciate my effort."

- **Inner Critic:** "I always mess things up. I'm not good at this."
  Reframe: "Mistakes are part of learning. Every time I try, I get better."

Interactive Activity: Reframing in Action

Throughout the week, notice when your inner critic shows up. Write down the negative thought, then practice reframing it. Reflect on how this exercise changes your perspective and reduces anxiety.

Building Resilience Through Action

Taking action, even imperfectly, is one of the most effective ways to combat perfectionism. Facing your fears directly diminishes their power and helps you build confidence over time.

- **Start Small:** Choose manageable tasks that allow you to experiment with letting go of perfection. For example, send an email without obsessing over every word, or share an idea in a meeting without rehearsing it repeatedly.

- **Embrace Incremental Progress:** Break larger tasks into smaller steps, focusing on completing one piece at a time. This reduces the pressure to produce a flawless result and allows you to celebrate small victories along the way.

Example:

A writer struggling with perfectionism might set a goal to write 500 words a day without editing. By focusing on the act of writing rather than the quality of the draft, they build momentum and overcome the paralysis of starting.

Interactive Activity: The "Good Enough" Experiment

1. Identify one task this week where you tend to overanalyze or avoid.
2. Commit to completing it with a focus on progress, not perfection.
3. Reflect on the experience:
    o What was the outcome?
    o How did it feel to release the need for perfection?
    o Did the task take less time or energy than usual?

Celebrating Imperfection

A key step in breaking the cycle of perfectionism is learning to value imperfection. Celebrate the effort and growth that come from trying, regardless of the outcome. Recognize that mistakes are opportunities to learn, not evidence of failure.

- **Reframe Mistakes:** Instead of viewing errors as shortcomings, see them as steps toward improvement.

- **Focus on Strengths:** Acknowledge what you did well in a task, even if it wasn't perfect.
- **Reward Progress:** Celebrate small wins, such as completing a challenging task or trying something new.

Example:

Imagine baking a cake that doesn't turn out as planned. Instead of focusing on the flaws, appreciate the effort you put into trying a new recipe and the joy of sharing it with others.

Interactive Activity: Imperfection Wins

At the end of each day, write down one "imperfect win." This could be something you tried for the first time, a mistake you learned from, or a task you completed without overthinking. Over time, you'll start to see the value in imperfection.

Creating a New Relationship with Fear

Fear often drives both perfectionism and avoidance. To break the cycle, it's important to develop a healthier relationship with fear.

- **Acknowledge Your Fear:** Recognize when fear is holding you back and name it. For example, "I'm afraid of being judged for this presentation."
- **Assess the Reality:** Ask yourself, "What's the worst that could happen?" Often, the feared outcome is less catastrophic than it feels.
- **Take Small Risks:** Gradually expose yourself to situations that trigger fear. Each time you face a fear and survive, you build resilience and confidence.

Example:

A perfectionist who avoids public speaking might start by presenting to a small, supportive group before moving on to larger audiences.

Over time, they'll realize they can handle criticism and mistakes, reducing their fear of failure.

Interactive Activity: Fear Inventory

1. Write down a list of fears that fuel your perfectionism.
2. For each fear, answer the following questions:
   - What am I afraid will happen?
   - How likely is that outcome?
   - What's a small step I can take to face this fear?
3. Commit to taking one small step this week and reflect on the experience.

Reflection Exercise: Your Progress Journey

Breaking the perfectionism-avoidance cycle is a process, and it's important to track your progress along the way. At the end of each week, spend time reflecting on the following prompts:

1. What tasks did I complete despite my perfectionist tendencies?
2. How did I reframe negative thoughts or fears this week?
3. What small steps did I take to face avoidance behaviors?
4. What did I learn from my imperfections or mistakes?

By consistently reflecting on your progress, you'll build self-awareness and momentum for continued growth. Over time, you'll find that progress—not perfection—becomes your new standard for success.

1.5 The Mental and Physical Costs of Perfection

The relentless pursuit of perfection may seem like a path to success, but it often comes at a steep price—one that affects not only your mental and physical health but also your relationships and overall quality of life. Understanding these costs is essential for taking meaningful steps toward change.

Mental Health Struggles

Perfectionism is strongly linked to a range of mental health challenges. The constant drive to meet unattainable standards creates a state of chronic stress, which can lead to:

- **Anxiety:** Perfectionists often experience excessive worry about outcomes, fueled by a fear of failure or judgment. This anxiety can make even simple tasks feel overwhelming.

- **Depression:** The inability to meet self-imposed or external standards can result in feelings of inadequacy, hopelessness, and despair. Over time, these emotions can spiral into clinical depression.

- **Obsessive-Compulsive Tendencies:** Perfectionists may develop repetitive thought patterns or behaviors in an attempt to maintain control. While these actions might provide temporary relief, they often perpetuate stress and dissatisfaction.

Example:

Imagine a student who rewrites the same paper multiple times, never feeling it's "good enough" to submit. They lose sleep, miss deadlines, and feel increasingly anxious and disheartened about their abilities.

Reflection Activity: Identifying Mental Health Impacts

Think about how perfectionism affects your mental health. In your journal, answer the following questions:

1. What emotions do you frequently experience when striving for perfection?

2. How does perfectionism influence your ability to relax or enjoy activities?

3. Are there specific situations where your perfectionist tendencies intensify feelings of stress or anxiety?

Physical Health Impacts

The mind and body are deeply interconnected, and the stress of perfectionism often manifests physically. Chronic stress caused by perfectionist tendencies can lead to:

- **Headaches:** Constant tension and overthinking can trigger frequent headaches or migraines.

- **Insomnia:** Perfectionists often replay their mistakes or unfinished tasks in their minds, making it difficult to wind down and fall asleep.

- **Digestive Issues:** Stress can disrupt the gut-brain connection, leading to stomachaches, nausea, or other gastrointestinal problems.

- **Weakened Immune System:** Chronic stress can suppress the immune system, which leaves perfectionists more susceptible to illnesses.

Example:

A professional who obsessively prepares for every meeting may skip meals, sacrifice sleep, and work through illness. Over time, these habits can result in burnout and significant health challenges.

Interactive Activity: Physical Health Check-In

Take a few minutes to assess how perfectionism affects your body. Answer these questions in your journal:

1. Do you notice any recurring physical symptoms during periods of high stress?

2. How does your body feel after a day of striving for perfection—tense, fatigued, or energized?

3. What physical changes do you observe when you give yourself permission to relax?

Social Isolation

Perfectionism doesn't only affect your internal well-being; it also shapes how you interact with others. The fear of judgment or failure can lead to:

- **Withdrawal:** Perfectionists may avoid social situations where they feel they can't meet expectations, leading to loneliness and isolation.

- **Strained Relationships:** Holding others to unrealistic standards can create tension and resentment in personal and professional relationships.

- **Missed Opportunities:** The reluctance to take risks or try new things for fear of failure can limit social and professional growth.

Example:

A perfectionist friend who declines invitations to gatherings because they worry about what to wear or how to behave may unintentionally distance themselves from their social circle, deepening feelings of isolation.

Reflection Activity: Social Impacts of Perfectionism

In your journal, explore the social costs of perfectionism:

1. Have you ever avoided social interactions because of fear of judgment or failure?

2. Do you feel your relationships are impacted by your high expectations—of yourself or others?

3. What steps can you take to prioritize connection over perfection in your social life?

Seeking Support

Breaking free from perfectionism is a journey, and sometimes professional support is essential. Therapy can provide tools and strategies to help you manage your perfectionist tendencies and improve your overall well-being.

- **Cognitive-Behavioral Therapy (CBT):** CBT helps perfectionists identify and challenge distorted thought patterns, replacing them with healthier, more balanced perspectives.

- **Mindfulness-Based Therapy:** Practicing mindfulness can teach you to live in the present moment, reducing overthinking and self-criticism.

- **Support Groups:** Joining a group of individuals facing similar struggles can provide a sense of connection and shared understanding.

Example:

A perfectionist seeking therapy learns to set realistic goals and embrace imperfection as part of growth. Over time, they experience reduced anxiety, improved self-esteem, and a greater sense of fulfillment.

Interactive Activity: Creating a Support Plan

1. Research local therapists or online therapy platforms specializing in perfectionism or anxiety.

2. List two or three strategies you've learned in this chapter that you can implement immediately.

3. Identify a trusted friend or family member who can support you as you work to manage perfectionism.

The Long-Term Effects of Ignoring Perfectionism

Without intervention, perfectionism's mental, physical, and social costs can compound over time. Chronic stress may lead to more serious health conditions like heart disease or autoimmune disorders. Relationships may suffer irreparable damage, and opportunities for personal and professional growth could be missed.

Reflection Exercise: Imagining a Healthier Future

Take a moment to visualize what your life might look like without the weight of perfectionism. In your journal, write about:

1. How would your mental and physical health improve?

2. What would your relationships look like?

3. What goals or dreams could you pursue if you weren't held back by the need to be perfect?

By recognizing the mental and physical costs of perfectionism, you take the first step toward reclaiming your health, happiness, and relationships. Change may not happen overnight, but with awareness and consistent effort, you can start to break free from perfectionism's grip and embrace a more balanced and fulfilling life.

1.6 Moving Toward Balance

Breaking free from perfectionism is a journey, not an overnight transformation. It's about shifting your mindset and habits step by step, learning to embrace progress over perfection, and finding fulfillment in the process rather than the end result. As you progress through this workbook, remember that even small changes can lead to significant growth. The goal isn't to abandon your drive for excellence but to approach it with self-compassion and balance.

Reevaluating Your Definition of Success

One of the most powerful steps in managing perfectionism is redefining what success looks like. For many perfectionists, success is tied to flawless execution, but this narrow definition often leads to burnout and dissatisfaction. Instead, consider broadening your perspective:

- **Focus on Growth:** Success isn't just about achieving a goal—it's about the lessons learned along the way. Celebrate your efforts, not just your outcomes.

- **Embrace Flexibility:** Perfectionists often rigidly stick to plans, but adaptability is a key component of success. Allow yourself to pivot when needed without viewing it as failure.

- **Prioritize Fulfillment:** Ask yourself if your goals align with your values and passions. True success comes from pursuing what brings you joy and meaning, not just external validation.

Activity: Redefining Success

In your journal, write down your current definition of success. Then, challenge yourself to reframe it with the following prompts:

1. What would success look like if it were based on personal growth rather than perfection?

2. How would you define success in a way that includes self-compassion and balance?

3. What small, achievable goals can you set that prioritize progress over perfection?

Cultivating Self-Compassion

Self-compassion is the antidote to the harsh self-criticism that fuels perfectionism. It involves treating yourself with the same kindness and understanding that you would offer a friend. When you make a mistake or fall short of your expectations, remind yourself that imperfection is part of being human.

Strategies to Build Self-Compassion:

- **Practice Positive Self-Talk:** Replace self-critical thoughts with affirming ones. For example, instead of saying, "I failed," say, "I tried my best, and that's enough."

- **Acknowledge Your Efforts:** Celebrate the work you've put in, even if the result isn't perfect. Effort is an accomplishment in itself.

- **Embrace Imperfection:** Remind yourself that everyone has flaws, and mistakes are opportunities for growth.

Example:

Imagine a chef who burns a dish while trying a new recipe. Instead of berating themselves, they focus on the fact that they took a creative risk and identify what they can do differently next time. This shift in perspective fosters resilience and encourages continued growth.

Building Healthy Habits

Creating new habits is essential for maintaining balance and preventing perfectionism from taking over. Focus on habits that promote well-being and reduce stress:

- **Set Boundaries:** Learn to say no to tasks or commitments that overwhelm you. Protecting your time and energy is crucial for maintaining balance.

- **Prioritize Self-Care:** Make time for activities that recharge you, whether it's exercise, meditation, reading, or spending time with loved ones.

- **Limit Overthinking:** Practice mindfulness to stay present and avoid spiraling into over analysis. Techniques like deep breathing or grounding exercises can help.

Activity: Habit Tracker

Create a weekly habit tracker in your journal. Choose three habits that support balance (e.g., setting boundaries, taking 10 minutes for mindfulness, or journaling). Check off each day you complete the habit and reflect on how these changes impact your stress levels and overall well-being.

Learning to Delegate

Perfectionists often struggle to delegate tasks, fearing they won't be done "right." However, delegation is a powerful way to reduce your workload and build trust in others.

- **Start Small:** Begin with tasks that feel less critical, like asking a colleague to proofread a document or having a family member help with household chores.

- **Communicate Clearly:** Provide clear instructions and trust others to follow through without micromanaging.

- **Accept Imperfection:** Recognize that others may not do things exactly as you would—and that's okay. The outcome is what matters, not the process.

Example:

A manager overwhelmed with reports learns to delegate sections of the work to their team. By trusting their colleagues and letting go of the need for perfection, they reduce their stress and foster collaboration.

Balancing Drive and Rest

Your ambition is a strength, but without balance, it can lead to exhaustion. Balancing drive with rest ensures that you can sustain your efforts without burning out.

- **Schedule Downtime:** Treat rest as a non-negotiable part of your schedule, just like work or errands.

- **Set Realistic Goals:** Break large tasks into smaller, manageable steps. Celebrate each milestone instead of waiting until the end to feel accomplished.

- **Know When to Step Back:** Pay attention to signs of burnout, such as irritability, fatigue, or loss of motivation. When you notice these signals, give yourself permission to take a break.

Interactive Activity: Creating a Balance Plan

In your journal, outline a weekly schedule that includes both work and rest. For each day, list one task or goal you want to accomplish and one way you'll prioritize rest (e.g., a 15-minute walk, an hour of reading, or a phone-free evening).

Visualizing a Balanced Future

Imagine what your life would look like without the weight of perfectionism. Visualizing your ideal balanced life can provide motivation and clarity as you work toward change.

Reflection Exercise: Your Ideal Day

Close your eyes and picture a day where perfectionism doesn't dictate your actions. Ask yourself:

1. How do you spend your time?
2. What emotions do you feel throughout the day?
3. How do you interact with others?

Write down your vision in detail. Use this as a guide to identify areas where you can make changes in your current routine to align with your ideal balanced life.

The Power of Gratitude

Gratitude can shift your focus from what's missing or imperfect to what's meaningful and fulfilling. Cultivating gratitude helps you appreciate progress, effort, and the people in your life.

Gratitude Practices:

- **Daily Gratitude Journal:** Write down three things you're grateful for each day. They can be as simple as a sunny morning or as significant as a personal achievement.

- **Express Appreciation:** Share your gratitude with others. Thank a colleague for their help, or tell a friend how much you value their support.

- **Focus on the Present:** Instead of dwelling on what could be better, take a moment to appreciate what is.

Example:

A perfectionist who always focuses on their to-do list starts a gratitude journal. Over time, they notice a shift in perspective, feeling more content with their accomplishments and less fixated on what's left undone.

By embracing these strategies, you can begin to move toward a life of balance and self-compassion. Progress won't happen all at once, but each small step brings you closer to breaking free from the grip of perfectionism and enjoying a more fulfilling, authentic life.

Embracing Self-Compassion

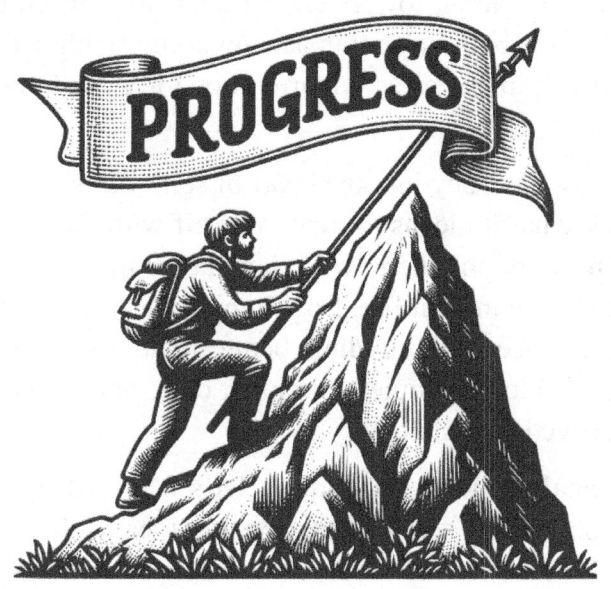

Visualize standing in front of a mirror. Instead of admiring the reflection of someone who's doing their best, your mind zeroes in on perceived flaws: a wrinkle here, a blemish there, a moment where you fell short today. The voice in your head doesn't just critique; it chastises, reminds, and replays. It whispers, "You're not enough."

Now, imagine if that voice spoke differently. What if, instead of criticism, it offered encouragement? What if, instead of dwelling on mistakes, it celebrated small victories? Picture it saying, "I see you're trying your best, and that's all anyone can ask." This is the shift that self-compassion invites—a powerful reframe of the way you speak to yourself.

For many of us, self-compassion feels like an alien concept. We're conditioned to believe that success requires relentless self-criticism, that toughness on ourselves is the only way to grow. We think offering ourselves kindness is indulgent or lazy. But here's the truth: self-compassion is not about lowering your standards or letting yourself off the hook. It's about balancing accountability with understanding. It's about seeing mistakes as opportunities for growth, not evidence of failure.

This chapter is a journey into the heart of self-compassion. Together, we'll unpack what it means to treat yourself with the same kindness and care you extend to others. We'll look at the transformative power of self-compassion in your life, from improving your mental health to fostering resilience and building better relationships. You'll also explore practical tools to quiet your inner critic and start cultivating a more supportive inner dialogue.

But before analyzing the techniques, let's acknowledge something important: practicing self-compassion isn't easy. If you've spent years—or decades—being your own harshest critic, shifting that narrative takes time, effort, and patience. And that's okay. Progress, not perfection, is the goal. As you work through this chapter, remember that self-compassion is not something you achieve; it's something you practice.

Let's start by understanding why self-compassion matters so much. The journey begins with a simple but profound truth: you are worthy of the same care and kindness you so freely give to others. Think about that for a moment. How would your life change if you treated yourself with even half the grace you extend to a friend? How much lighter would your days feel if, instead of replaying mistakes, you embraced them as part of the learning process?

The Struggle of Self-Compassion

It is worth reflecting on why self-compassion can feel so elusive. For many of us, it's not just about what we think of ourselves—it's about the messages we've absorbed from the world around us.

Cultural Conditioning

In a world that values hustle and perfection, self-compassion can feel counterintuitive. We're bombarded with messages that equate worth with achievement: the perfect career, the perfect family, the perfect life. Social media amplifies this pressure, offering carefully curated glimpses into other people's seemingly flawless realities.

The Inner Critic as a Protector

Your inner critic didn't develop overnight. For most of us, it started as a defense mechanism. Maybe it was a way to anticipate criticism from others and avoid disappointment. Maybe it was a misguided attempt to motivate ourselves to do better. Over time, though, the inner critic becomes less of a coach and more of a tyrant, leaving us feeling exhausted and unworthy.

The Fear of Self-Compassion

Here's a paradox: even though self-compassion feels good, it can also feel risky. If you've relied on self-criticism to drive your success, letting go of that habit might feel like losing your edge. But here's the reality: self-compassion doesn't weaken you—it strengthens you. It allows you to recover more quickly from setbacks, approach challenges with clarity, and maintain a healthier perspective.

Why This Chapter Matters

The tools and exercises in this chapter are more than just strategies—they're invitations to reimagine your relationship with yourself. You'll learn how to:

- Quiet the voice of your inner critic without losing accountability.
- Build daily habits that reinforce kindness, mindfulness, and connection.
- Recognize self-compassion as a strength, not a weakness.

By the end of this chapter, you'll have a deeper understanding of what self-compassion looks like in practice and how it can transform the way you navigate life's challenges.

2.1 What is Self-Compassion?

Self-compassion, as defined by Dr. Kristin Neff, is a practice of extending the same kindness, understanding, and care to yourself that you would offer to a loved one. It's not about letting yourself off the hook or lowering your standards. Instead, self-compassion is about finding balance—acknowledging your imperfections while still holding yourself accountable for growth. Let's review the three foundational pillars of self-compassion and explore their profound impact on our lives.

Three Core Elements of Self-Compassion

1. Self-Kindness vs. Self-Judgment

Imagine your best friend comes to you after making a mistake at work. They feel terrible and are beating themselves up over it. Would you scold them and say, "You're a failure"? Of course not! You'd likely reassure them, saying something like, "Mistakes happen. You'll learn from this."

Self-kindness is about offering yourself that same care. It involves replacing harsh self-criticism with understanding and empathy. Instead of berating yourself for falling short, you can acknowledge the effort you made and recognize that imperfection is a part of being human.

Case Study:

Amy, a graduate student, struggled with self-criticism after receiving feedback on a research paper. Her advisor highlighted areas for improvement, and Amy spiraled into negative self-talk: "I'm terrible at this. I'll never finish my thesis." Through practicing self-kindness, Amy reframed her inner dialogue. She reminded herself that feedback was a tool for growth, not a condemnation of her abilities. By shifting her perspective, she felt more confident tackling revisions and completed her thesis with pride.

Exercise: Self-Kindness Letter

Write a letter to yourself about a recent challenge. Pretend you're writing to a friend, offering encouragement and understanding. What would you say to lift them up? Save the letter and revisit it when you need a reminder to be kind to yourself.

2. Common Humanity vs. Isolation

When you're facing a setback, it's easy to feel like you're the only one struggling. Self-compassion reminds us that suffering is a universal experience. Everyone makes mistakes, experiences failures, and has bad days. Recognizing this shared humanity fosters connection and reduces feelings of isolation.

Example:

Consider Maya, who was passed over for a promotion. Initially, she felt inadequate and alone, assuming her colleagues were excelling while she lagged behind. By reflecting on common humanity, she realized that many of her peers had also faced professional setbacks. This awareness helped her view her experience as part of the larger human story, not as a personal failing.

Activity: Shared Struggles List

Make a list of people you admire—friends, family, or public figures. Next to each name, write one struggle or mistake they've openly shared. Reflect on how these challenges shaped their growth. This exercise reinforces the idea that imperfection is universal and not a reflection of your worth.

3. Mindfulness vs. Over-Identification

Mindfulness is the ability to observe your thoughts and emotions without becoming consumed by them. It's about acknowledging what you're feeling—whether it's sadness, anger, or frustration—without letting those emotions define you.

When you over-identify with negative thoughts, you risk getting stuck in a cycle of rumination. Mindfulness offers a way out by creating space between you and your inner experiences.

Case Study:

James, an entrepreneur, often felt overwhelmed by anxiety during high-pressure meetings. Instead of spiraling into self-doubt, he started practicing mindfulness. Before each meeting, he took a few minutes to focus on his breath, grounding himself in the present moment. During the meeting, he reminded himself, "This is just anxiety. It doesn't control me." Over time, this practice helped him stay calm and perform better.

Mindfulness Exercise:

- Sit in a quiet place and close your eyes.

- Take slow, deep breaths, focusing on the sensation of the air entering and leaving your body.

- When a negative thought arises, label it (e.g., "That's self-doubt") and let it pass without judgment. Return focus to your breath.
  Practice this for 5-10 minutes daily to build mindfulness skills.

Addressing Common Misconceptions About Self-Compassion

Self-compassion is often misunderstood as self-indulgence or weakness. These misconceptions can prevent people from embracing its benefits.

Myth: Self-Compassion Is Self-Indulgence

Reality: Self-compassion doesn't mean ignoring responsibilities or avoiding growth. It's about addressing mistakes constructively without unnecessary self-punishment.

Myth: Self-Compassion Is Weakness

Reality: It takes strength to confront your struggles with honesty and kindness. Self-compassion builds resilience, helping you bounce back from setbacks more effectively.

Exercise: Myth-Busting Reflection

Reflect on any beliefs you hold about self-compassion. Are there misconceptions that prevent you from practicing it? Write down these beliefs and challenge them with evidence or examples from your life.

Building a Foundation for Self-Compassion

The three pillars of self-compassion—self-kindness, common humanity, and mindfulness—offer a roadmap for transforming your relationship with yourself. They're not just abstract concepts; they're practical tools you can integrate into daily life.

To get started, choose one pillar to focus on this week. Whether it's practicing mindfulness, reaching out to someone to share a struggle, or writing a self-kindness letter, these small steps can create meaningful change over time.

Interactive Worksheet: The Self-Compassion Check-In

Download a worksheet that helps you track daily acts of self-compassion. For each day, note:

- A moment when you practiced self-kindness.

- A situation where you reminded yourself of shared humanity.

- A time when you used mindfulness to manage a challenging emotion.

By the end of the week, review your check-in to celebrate your progress and identify areas for growth.

2.3 Techniques for Cultivating Self-Compassion

Practicing self-compassion requires intention and commitment, but the rewards are transformative. Below, we expand on foundational techniques such as self-compassionate letter writing, daily affirmations, and loving-kindness meditation, adding depth, examples, and interactive exercises to help you embrace kindness and understanding toward yourself.

Self-Compassionate Letter Writing

Writing a self-compassionate letter is a therapeutic exercise that allows you to address your struggles with empathy and kindness. Instead of dwelling on your perceived shortcomings, this activity helps you reframe challenges and celebrate your resilience.

How to Begin:

1. Start by identifying a specific situation where you felt you fell short.

2. Write about the emotions you experienced, as though you're talking to a dear friend who is going through the same challenge.

3. Highlight your strengths, efforts, and areas of growth.

Case Study:

Rachel, a working mom, felt immense guilt for missing her son's soccer game due to a work deadline. In her letter, she acknowledged her disappointment but also celebrated her dedication to providing for her family. She wrote:

"I know you feel like you let him down but remember how much you're doing to create opportunities for your family. You're not perfect, and that's okay. You're showing him resilience and balance in real life."

By the end of the exercise, Rachel felt a sense of relief and was better equipped to approach her day with clarity and self-acceptance.

Interactive Activity:

Write a self-compassionate letter this week. Set a timer for 15 minutes and write without stopping. Keep it in a journal or revisit it when self-doubt creeps in.

Daily Affirmations

Affirmations are more than just positive words; they are tools to rewire your thought patterns and cultivate a nurturing inner voice. The key is consistency and personal relevance.

How to Use Them:

- Select affirmations that resonate with your current struggles or goals.
- Speak them aloud each morning or write them in your journal.
- Incorporate them into your daily routine by placing them on sticky notes around your home or setting reminders on your phone.

Examples of Affirmations:

- "I am a work in progress, and progress is enough."
- "My value is not tied to my productivity."
- "I deserve kindness, especially from myself."

Case Study:

Liam, a recent college graduate, struggled with imposter syndrome in his new job. He wrote affirmations on sticky notes and placed them on his bathroom mirror:

- "I belong here."

- "I am capable of learning and growing."
  Repeating these daily helped Liam shift his perspective and approach his work with more confidence.

Interactive Activity:

Choose three affirmations to focus on this week. Record yourself saying them and play the recording during moments of stress or self-doubt. Hearing your own voice can amplify their impact.

Loving-Kindness Mediation

This mindfulness practice fosters compassion for yourself and others, creating a ripple effect of empathy and peace.

How to Practice:

1. Sit in a quiet space and close your eyes.

2. Begin by focusing on your breath.

3. Repeat the following phrases silently or aloud:

    o "May I be happy."

    o "May I be healthy."

    o "May I be safe."

    o "May I be at peace."

4. Begin by extending these positive intentions to loved ones, then gradually include acquaintances and even individuals with whom you've had disagreements.

Case Study:

Liz, a teacher, often felt overwhelmed by her students' demands. Through loving-kindness meditation, she began each day by sending compassionate thoughts to herself and her class:

"May I have patience today. May my students feel supported. May we all grow together."

This practice transformed her perspective, reducing stress and fostering a positive classroom environment.

Interactive Activity:

Set aside five minutes each day for loving-kindness meditation. Use a guided meditation app or create your own script to follow. Afterward, journal your reflections on how it made you feel.

Visualization Exercises

Visualization is a powerful tool to help you mentally rehearse self-compassion in challenging situations.

How to Practice:

- Close your eyes and imagine yourself in a stressful situation, like receiving constructive feedback.
- Visualize yourself responding with kindness and understanding. Instead of self-criticism, imagine saying, "I'm learning, and this is part of the process."
- Picture yourself feeling calm and centered, navigating the situation with confidence.

Case Study:

During team meetings, Jordan, a manager, often felt the need to have all the answers. Through visualization, he practiced responding with phrases like, "That's a great question—I'll look into it and follow up." By mentally rehearsing this response, he felt less pressure to be perfect and more focused on collaboration.

Interactive Activity:

Create a "visualization diary." After each visualization session, write down what you imagined and how it made you feel. Reflect on how this exercise might influence your actions in real-life scenarios.

Develop a Self-Compassion Routine

Incorporating self-compassion into your daily routine ensures it becomes a habit rather than an occasional practice.

Morning Ritual:

- Begin with a mindfulness exercise or affirmation.

- Set an intention for the day: "Today, I will approach myself with kindness, no matter what."

Midday Check-In:

- Pause during your lunch break to reflect: "How am I treating myself today? Am I being kind and supportive?"

Evening Reflection:

- Journal about one moment where you showed yourself compassion and one area where you could improve.

Case Study:

Samantha, a busy entrepreneur, felt she had no time for self-care. She started a simple routine: reciting an affirmation while brushing her teeth in the morning and journaling for five minutes before bed. These small acts created a sense of balance and mindfulness that improved her overall well-being.

Group or Partner Exercises

Practicing self-compassion doesn't have to be a solo journey. Engaging with a friend or support group can deepen your practice.

Activity: Compassion Buddy Check-Ins

- Partner with a friend and schedule weekly check-ins.

- Share one moment of self-compassion from your week and one area where you struggled.

- Offer each other encouragement and ideas for improvement.

Case Study:

Leah and her coworker, Ben, formed a self-compassion accountability partnership. During weekly coffee chats, they discussed their progress and shared strategies, like using affirmations or reframing negative thoughts. This mutual support helped both of them stay committed to their goals.

By incorporating these techniques, exercises, and activities into your life, you'll create a foundation for self-compassion that grows stronger with practice. Over time, these habits will become second nature, transforming the way you treat yourself and navigate challenges. Remember, self-compassion is not a destination but an ongoing journey—one that can lead to profound growth and inner peace.

2.4 Transforming the Inner Critic

The inner critic, often born from past experiences and external pressures, can be relentless in its pursuit of perfection. It distorts reality, undermines confidence, and fuels self-doubt. However, with conscious effort and practical techniques, you can transform this internal adversary into a supportive guide. This section explores tools and strategies to reshape the inner critic's voice, providing case studies, examples, and exercises to help you break free from its grip.

Understanding the Inner Critic

The inner critic operates as a defense mechanism, attempting to protect you from failure or rejection. However, its harshness often does more harm than good. Recognizing its origins is the first step toward change. Reflect on the following:

- Where Reflect on the origins of this critical voice. Could it have been influenced by early life experiences, cultural pressures, or previous setbacks?

- What does your inner critic sound like? Does it mimic a parent, teacher, or someone else from your past?

Case Study:

Emily's inner critic mirrored her high school coach's voice, who often said, "If you're not the best, why bother?" This belief followed her into adulthood, leaving her paralyzed by the fear of not excelling. By identifying the source, Emily began to question its validity and reframe her thoughts.

Reframing Negative Thoughts

One of the most effective ways to transform the inner critic is to challenge its negative narratives with constructive alternatives.

Steps to Reframing Negative Thoughts:

1. Recognize the Thought: Catch yourself in the moment. For example, "I always mess things up."

2. Challenge the Thought: Consider asking yourself, "Is this completely accurate?" or "What proof do I have to back this up?"

3. Reframe the Thought: Replace it with a kinder perspective, such as, "I made a mistake, but mistakes are part of learning."

Example:

- Negative Thought: "I'll never be good at this."
- Reframed Thought: "I'm learning, and every attempt brings me closer to improvement."

Interactive Activity:

Create a "Thought Transformation Journal." Dedicate a page each day to record:

- The negative thought.

- The situation or trigger.

- A reframed, constructive alternative. Over time, observe patterns and celebrate moments when reframing felt natural.

Cognitive Restructuring

Cognitive restructuring, a technique from cognitive-behavioral therapy (CBT), involves reshaping distorted thoughts to align with reality.

Steps to Cognitive Restructuring:

1. Identify the Distortion: Is the thought a generalization, catastrophic prediction, or an all-or-nothing statement?

2. Challenge the Thought: Ask, "What would I say to a friend thinking this way?"

3. Replace with Realistic Thinking: Shift to a balanced perspective.

Example:

- Distorted Thought: "If I don't finish this project perfectly, my career is over."

- Balanced Thought: "Completing this project is important, but one outcome doesn't define my career."

Case Study:

Jake, a graphic designer, often delayed starting projects due to his fear of imperfection. By practicing cognitive restructuring, he reframed his thoughts: "Starting imperfectly is better than not starting at all." This shift helped him meet deadlines with less anxiety.

Interactive Activity:

Use a chart to practice restructuring:

Negative Thought	Evidence Supporting It	Evidence Against It	Balanced Perspective
"I am terrible at public speaking".	"I stumbled during a presentation".	"My last talk received positive feedback."	"I can improve with practice."

Building Self-Awareness

The inner critic often operates in the background, unnoticed. Building self-awareness helps you recognize its presence and take control.

Mindfulness Techniques:

- Pause and Observe: When a critical thought arises, take a moment to breathe and observe it without judgment.
- Name the Critic: Assign a name or persona to your inner critic to distance yourself from it. For instance, call it "Judge Jerry" or "Critical Chris." This helps you see it as a separate entity rather than an inherent part of yourself.

Case Study:

Kelly named her inner critic "The Perfectionist." When she noticed self-critical thoughts, she would say, "Thanks for your input, Perfectionist, but I've got this." This lighthearted approach made it easier to challenge the critic's influence.

Practical Exercises

1. Inner Critic Audit

At the end of each day, jot down instances when your inner critic appeared. Reflect on:

- The situation.

- What the critic said.

- How you responded. This exercise increases awareness and helps you identify triggers.

2. Compassionate Response Practice

Write a dialogue between your inner critic and your compassionate self.

- Critic: "You'll never succeed at this."

- Compassionate Self: "I might stumble, but I'm learning and growing every step of the way."

3. Visualization Exercise

Visualize your inner critic as a character. What does it look like? Is it stern, disapproving, or frantic? Now, imagine shrinking this character and placing it in a jar. This visualization diminishes its power and reminds you that you're in control.

Interactive Reflection Exercise

Reflect on your relationship with your inner critic using these prompts:

1. What phrases does your inner critic use most often?

2. What situations trigger your critic's voice?

3. How can you reframe those phrases into compassionate, constructive thoughts?

Write down your reflections and revisit them regularly.

Transforming your inner critic is not about silencing it entirely but learning to engage with it constructively. By practicing these techniques, you'll develop a more compassionate inner dialogue, paving the way for growth, resilience, and self-acceptance. With time, you'll find that the voice of your critic becomes softer, replaced by a kind and encouraging guide.

2.5 Mindful Moments of Self-Compassion

Bringing mindfulness and self-compassion into routine tasks helps anchor these practices into your day. Small, intentional actions can have a profound impact over time.

Examples of Mindful Moments:

1. Brushing Your Teeth: As you brush, take a moment to reflect on one thing you appreciate about yourself. For example, "I'm proud of how I handled today's challenges."

2. Morning Coffee or Tea: While sipping your drink, set an intention for the day that prioritizes self-kindness, such as, "I will be patient with myself today."

3. Commuting: Whether you're driving, walking, or taking public transportation, silently repeat a mantra like, "I am enough" or "I'm doing the best I can."

Case Study:

Anna, a high school teacher, found her mornings chaotic and stressful. By turning her commute into a time for mindfulness, she began repeating affirmations while driving. This simple habit helped her start each day with a calmer and more positive mindset.

Compassionate Boundaries

Establishing boundaries is a meaningful expression of self-respect and an essential way to nurture self-compassion. Boundaries help protect your time, energy, and emotional well-being.

Steps to Setting Compassionate Boundaries:

1. Identify Your Limits: Reflect on situations where you feel overwhelmed or stretched too thin. These are areas where boundaries are needed.

2. Communicate clearly and kindly: For instance, you might say: "Thank you for thinking of me, but I need to prioritize my current responsibilities."

3. Prioritize Your Needs: Remember that saying "no" to others is saying "yes" to yourself.

Example:

David, a software engineer, often felt burned out because he struggled to say no to extra work. By setting a boundary that limited overtime hours, he regained his evenings for rest and personal growth.

Interactive Activity:

Write down one area in your life where you need stronger boundaries. Practice scripting a response for setting that boundary kindly but firmly. For example:

- Situation: A friend frequently asks for last-minute favors.

- Boundary Script: "I care about helping you, but I need more notice to fit it into my schedule."

Evening Gratitude Practice

Ending your day with gratitude for acts of self-compassion reinforces the habit and creates a positive mindset for the following day.

How to Practice Evening Gratitude:

1. Reflect on Acts of Kindness: Before bed, think of three ways you were kind to yourself during the day. These could be small actions, such as taking a break or reframing a critical thought.

2. Note How It Felt: Reflect on how those acts of kindness impacted your mood or energy.

3. Plan for Tomorrow: Identify one way you'll continue practicing self-compassion the next day.

Case Study:

Sophia, a small business owner, started journaling three self-kind acts each evening. Over time, this practice helped her notice and celebrate her progress, reducing feelings of self-doubt.

Practical Examples of Self-Compassion in Action

1. Approaching Mistakes with Kindness

Instead of criticizing yourself for errors, view them as opportunities for growth.

Example: If you miss a deadline, remind yourself: "This is a chance to reassess my priorities and improve my time management."

2. Allowing Yourself to Rest

Recognize that rest is a vital part of self-care, not a sign of laziness.

Example: If you're feeling overwhelmed, take a 15-minute break without guilt, knowing it will recharge your focus and energy.

3. Celebrating Small Wins

Acknowledge and celebrate even minor achievements. Example: If you complete a challenging task, reward yourself with a small treat or simply take a moment to appreciate your effort.

Interactive Activity:

Create a "Small Wins Journal." Each evening, jot down one thing you accomplished and how you showed kindness to yourself in the process.

Case Study: Turning Self-Compassion Into a Habit

Take a moment to reflect on your own journey with self-compassion. Have you ever noticed how small, consistent changes in your behavior can lead to significant shifts over time? The following example illustrates how one person embraced self-compassion and transformed their daily life. As you read Rebecca's story, think about parallels in your own experience and how her strategies might inspire your next steps.

Name: Rebecca

Challenge: Rebecca, a marketing professional, struggled with perfectionism and often criticized herself for not meeting her high standards.

Action Plan: Rebecca implemented a daily gratitude practice, set boundaries with her workload, and started using affirmations during her morning routine.

Outcome: Over six months, Rebecca noticed a significant decrease in her stress levels and an improvement in her overall happiness. By integrating self-compassion into her daily life, she felt more balanced and confident.

2.6 Myths About Self-Compassion

Self-compassion often suffers from a public relations problem, misunderstood as a sign of weakness, self-indulgence, or an excuse to avoid responsibility. These misconceptions can discourage individuals from embracing it fully, fearing that being kind to themselves may lead to complacency or mediocrity. In truth, self-compassion is a powerful and transformative practice that fosters accountability, resilience, and personal growth. Let's explore some of the common myths about self-compassion and unravel the truth behind them.

Myth 1: Self-Compassion Is Self-Indulgence

A common misperception is that practicing self-compassion means letting yourself off the hook or indulging in unproductive behaviors. For example, some might believe that being kind to yourself equates to eating an entire tub of ice cream after a stressful day or binge-watching TV instead of addressing responsibilities. While occasional treats and relaxation can be part of self-care, self-compassion is much deeper. It's about acknowledging your struggles without self-judgment and making choices that truly support your well-being in the long run.

True self-compassion asks: *What do I really need in this moment to take care of myself?* Sometimes, the answer might be rest, and other times, it might mean pushing forward in a gentler, more mindful way. Far from enabling laziness, self-compassion provides the mental clarity to assess what actions will genuinely serve your growth and happiness.

Myth 2: Self-Compassion Leads to Laziness or Lower Standards

Another myth is that self-compassion will make you lose your drive or ambition. For perfectionists especially, the fear of lowering their high standards can feel unsettling. However, research shows that self-compassion actually enhances motivation and performance. By reducing the fear of failure, it creates a safer space to take risks, try new things, and persist through challenges.

For example, imagine two students preparing for an important exam. One berates themselves for every incorrect answer, while the other acknowledges mistakes as opportunities for improvement. The second student is likely to approach their studies with greater focus and less burnout because they're not weighed down by self-criticism. Self-compassion doesn't mean you stop striving for excellence—it means you approach goals with encouragement rather than fear, which often leads to better outcomes.

Myth 3: Self-Compassion Is Weakness

In a world that often values toughness and stoicism, self-compassion can mistakenly be seen as a vulnerability. Yet, it takes immense strength to face your shortcomings with honesty and kindness rather than denial or self-criticism. Self-compassion builds emotional resilience, enabling you to recover from setbacks more quickly and approach challenges with a clear, balanced mindset.

Consider how you would view a friend who demonstrates kindness and patience toward themselves after a failure. You'd likely admire their strength and emotional intelligence, recognizing that these traits allow them to grow rather than be consumed by guilt or shame. Practicing self-compassion for yourself requires the same courage and wisdom—it's not a sign of weakness but a reflection of inner strength.

Myth 4: Self-Compassion Is Selfish

Some people worry that focusing on their own needs will take attention away from others. In reality, self-compassion equips you to be more present and effective in your relationships. When you take the time to care for yourself, you have more emotional energy to support those around you. Think of it like the oxygen mask rule on an airplane: you must secure your own mask before assisting others.

By nurturing your own well-being, you're better able to show up for your loved ones with patience, empathy, and understanding. Self-compassion allows you to set healthy boundaries, preventing burnout and ensuring that your acts of kindness come from a place of genuine care rather than obligation or depletion.

Myth 5: Self-Compassion Means Avoiding Responsibility

One of the most pervasive myths is that self-compassion involves ignoring mistakes or refusing to take responsibility for your actions. This couldn't be further from the truth. Self-compassion encourages accountability without the harsh self-judgment that can lead to shame and defensiveness. Instead of dwelling on what went wrong, self-compassion helps you focus on what you can learn and how you can grow.

For instance, if you miss a deadline at work, self-compassion might sound like this: *"I made a mistake, but I'm human, and mistakes happen. I'll apologize, take steps to fix it, and reflect on how to improve my time management moving forward."* This balanced approach fosters both personal growth and professional integrity, proving that self-compassion and responsibility go hand in hand.

Embracing self-compassion requires challenging these myths and reframing your perspective. It's not about taking the easy way out or excusing poor behavior; it's about treating yourself with the understanding and care that empowers you to face life's challenges with resilience and grace. By dismantling these misconceptions, you can fully embrace self-compassion as a tool for personal growth, emotional well-being, and stronger connections with those around you.

Emotional Resilience and Flexibility

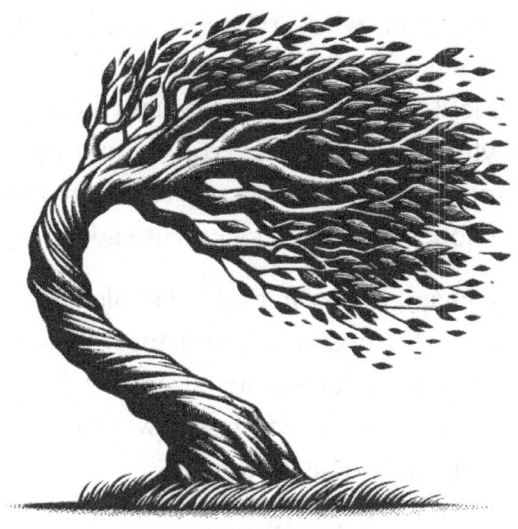

Imagine standing in the eye of a storm, where chaos swirls around you. The winds howl, the rain lashes down, yet amidst the turmoil, you find an unexpected stillness within yourself. This inner calm, even when everything around you may seem uncertain or overwhelming, is the hallmark of emotional resilience. Emotional resilience is the ability to navigate through life's inevitable challenges with strength, adaptability, and determination. It's not about pretending hardships don't exist or avoiding them altogether—it's about facing them head-on and learning to thrive despite them.

Resilience doesn't mean suppressing emotions or enduring difficulties without support. Instead, it involves recognizing challenges, processing your feelings, and choosing how to respond in a way that aligns with your values and goals. Think of resilience as a muscle—it grows stronger through practice, intentional effort, and the experiences that test it. Cultivating this ability equips you to recover from setbacks, persist through difficulties, and continue moving forward, even when the path ahead seems uncertain.

In today's fast-paced and unpredictable world, emotional resilience is not just a luxury; it's a necessity. Every day presents new challenges, whether they come from work, relationships, health, or unexpected changes. Stress is a constant companion for many, but resilience acts as a protective shield, allowing you to process these pressures without becoming overwhelmed. It enables you to find moments of clarity amidst confusion, to pause and reflect instead of reacting impulsively, and to hold onto hope even when faced with adversity.

Throughout this chapter, you'll find relatable examples, reflection exercises, and actionable tips to help you apply these concepts in your life. The goal is not to eliminate stress or hardship—they are inevitable parts of life—but to equip you with the tools to face them with grace, strength, and adaptability.

3.1 Building Emotional Resilience

Emotional resilience isn't something you're simply born with—it's a skill you can develop and refine over time. Think of it as an internal toolkit that helps you adapt, recover, and grow in the face of adversity. Resilience allows you to navigate challenges with clarity and strength, transforming what might feel like insurmountable obstacles into opportunities for personal growth and self-discovery.

This section explores key strategies for building emotional resilience, offering tools and insights to help you thrive through life's inevitable ups and downs. By embracing these techniques, you'll learn to view challenges not as setbacks but as milestones on your journey toward greater strength and self-awareness.

A Mindset Shift: Turning Obstacles into Opportunities

At the heart of emotional resilience lies a positive outlook. It's about reframing challenges as opportunities for growth rather than as insurmountable barriers. Instead of asking, "Why is this happening to me?" ask, "What can I learn from this experience?" This shift in perspective transforms obstacles into stages for personal development.

For example, consider Emma, a graphic designer who faced unexpected job loss. Initially overwhelmed by self-doubt, she decided to view the setback as an opportunity to pursue freelance work. By taking courses to sharpen her skills and networking within her industry, Emma not only rebuilt her career but also discovered a passion for entrepreneurship. Her resilience allowed her to turn adversity into a launchpad for success.

Emotional Regulation Techniques

Emotional regulation is the cornerstone of resilience. By learning to manage your emotions effectively, you gain control over how you respond to stress. Key techniques include:

- **Deep Breathing:** When emotions run high, pause and take slow, deep breaths. This simple practice calms your nervous system, reducing anxiety and helping you regain focus.

- **Mindfulness:** Cultivate awareness of the present moment without judgment. Mindfulness practices, such as meditation or body scans, help you observe your emotions with clarity and prevent them from overwhelming you.

- **Cognitive Reframing:** Challenge negative thoughts by examining their validity. Replace catastrophic thinking with balanced perspectives. For instance, instead of thinking, "I'll never succeed," tell yourself, "This is a setback, not a failure. I can learn and improve."

Gratitude as a Resilience Tool

Gratitude practices foster positivity and strengthen emotional resilience. Regularly acknowledging the good in your life helps shift your focus from what's lacking to what's present. Start a gratitude journal and jot down three things you're thankful for each day. Over time, this practice rewires your brain to notice and appreciate positive experiences, building a more resilient mindset.

Social Support: Building Your Network

Strong relationships are a critical component of emotional resilience. Having a network of supportive friends, family, and mentors creates a strong foundation to lean on during difficult times. These connections offer empathy, perspective, and encouragement, helping you navigate adversity with greater confidence.

Interactive Activity: Building a Support Network

Purpose: Identify and strengthen relationships that contribute to your resilience.

Instructions:

1. Draw a **Support Network Web** with your name in the center.

2. Add branches for different types of support, such as:

    o Emotional (friends, family)

    o Practical (mentors, colleagues)

    o Inspirational (books, podcasts, role models)

3. Write down the names of specific people or resources in each category.

4. Set an action plan to connect with at least one person or resource each week. For example:

    o Call a supportive friend for a catch-up.

    o Schedule time with a mentor to discuss goals.

    o Listen to an inspiring podcast during your commute.

3.2 Flexibility: Adapting to Change

Flexibility is like a tree bending in the wind. Its strength doesn't lie in resisting the force but in adapting to it. In today's dynamic world, adaptability has become a cornerstone of success. Whether it's a career shift, personal challenges, or unexpected disruptions like a global pandemic, those who embrace change are better equipped to thrive. Flexibility empowers you to face uncertainty with resilience, finding opportunities in the unexpected.

Cultivating Mental Flexibility

Building mental flexibility requires intentional practice. It's about training your mind to shift perspectives, think creatively, and respond calmly to change. Here's how to start:

1. Brainstorming Sessions

Encourage divergent thinking by exploring multiple solutions to a problem. For example, if you're struggling with time management, brainstorm five different ways to reorganize your schedule. This practice fosters creativity and helps you consider alternative approaches.

2. Role-Playing Scenarios

Simulate challenging situations to practice adapting in real-time. For instance, imagine a scenario where a major project deadline is moved up unexpectedly. Act out how you would reprioritize tasks, communicate with your team, and manage stress. This exercise helps you prepare for high-pressure situations and strengthens your adaptability.

3. Perspective-Shifting Exercises

Challenge yourself to view situations from different angles. For example:

- **Your Perspective:** "This change is overwhelming."

- **Another's Perspective:** "This is an exciting opportunity for innovation."
- **Neutral Perspective:** "This is a shift that requires adjustment."
  This reframing technique helps you break out of rigid thought patterns.

Embracing Uncertainty

Uncertainty often feels like a storm cloud hovering overhead, but it doesn't have to be paralyzing. By embracing ambiguity, you can turn fear into opportunity. Start by focusing on what you can control and letting go of the rest.

Journaling for Clarity

Reflect on past experiences where you successfully navigated uncertainty:

- What actions did you take to adapt?
- What lessons did you learn from the experience?
  Write about these moments to remind yourself of your ability to handle change.

Mindfulness in Uncertainty

Practice mindfulness exercises to stay grounded in the present moment:

- **Body Scan Meditation:** Close your eyes and focus on the sensations in each part of your body, starting from your toes and moving upward. This exercise helps reduce anxiety tied to uncertainty.

- **Acceptance Affirmations:** Repeat phrases like, "I accept what I cannot control and focus on what I can." These affirmations build a sense of inner peace amidst ambiguity.

Setting Flexible Goals

Rigid, unchangeable goals can feel like anchors dragging you down when circumstances shift. Instead, aim for adaptable goals that allow room for change while keeping you focused on your destination.

1. Create a Goal Map

Visualize your goal as a destination and chart multiple paths to get there. For example:

- Goal: "Save $5,000 in six months."
- Paths:
    - Cut discretionary spending.
    - Take on freelance work.
    - Sell unused items online.

        If one path becomes blocked, you have alternatives to keep moving forward.

2. Develop Contingency Plans

For each goal, identify potential obstacles and brainstorm solutions in advance. For example:

- **Obstacle:** "Unexpected car repair expenses."
- **Solution:** "Pause savings for one month and increase freelance work hours."
    Knowing you have backup plans reduces stress and increases confidence in your ability to adapt.

4. Celebrate Progress, Not Perfection
    Recognize that progress is more important than perfection. Adaptable goals allow you to adjust timelines and methods without feeling like you've failed. For example, if your workout goal shifts from running five days a week to three, celebrate the consistency rather than fixating on the change.

Interactive Activities

Activity 1: Flexibility Brainstorm

Write down a current challenge you're facing. Then, brainstorm three alternative ways to approach it. For example:

- **Challenge:** "I'm struggling to balance work and family."
- **Solutions:**
    - Schedule dedicated family time during weekends.
    - Use time-blocking techniques to create work-life boundaries.
    - Delegate tasks at work or home to free up time.

Activity 2: The Change Journal

Create a journal dedicated to reflecting on change:

- Write about one change you're currently experiencing.
- List what aspects of the change are within your control and what are not.
- Brainstorm actions you can take to adapt to the controllable aspects.

Activity 3: Flexibility Challenge

For one week, intentionally make small changes to your routine:

- Take a different route to work.
- Try a new food or recipe.
- Alter your workout schedule.

    At the end of the week, reflect on how these small changes made you feel. Did they boost your confidence in adapting to bigger shifts?

Flexibility is not about surrendering control—it's about recalibrating your approach to navigate life's unpredictability. By cultivating mental flexibility, embracing uncertainty, and setting adaptable goals, you equip yourself to turn challenges into opportunities for growth. As you practice these techniques, you'll find that change becomes less intimidating and more empowering.

3.3 Constructive Responses to Criticism

Criticism is an inevitable part of life, and how we process and respond to it defines its impact on our growth. While it can sting at first, criticism often offers insights we may not have seen ourselves. By learning to reframe feedback, filter out unhelpful comments, and embrace constructive suggestions, you can transform criticism into a powerful tool for self-betterment. This section explores how to approach criticism with curiosity and grace to foster personal and professional development.

Reframing Feedback

Criticism doesn't have to be a stumbling block; it can be a stepping stone to growth. The key is shifting your mindset to see feedback as an opportunity rather than a threat. When you reframe criticism, you unlock its potential to drive self-improvement.

Consider Sandra, a project manager who was told her reports were too detailed and hard to follow. At first, she felt defensive, but she decided to view the feedback as a chance to refine her communication skills. By simplifying her reports and focusing on clarity, Sandra not only improved her work but also earned greater respect from her colleagues. This transformation was made possible by approaching criticism as a learning tool rather than a judgment.

Understanding Types of Criticism

Not all feedback is created equal and understanding the difference between constructive and destructive criticism is essential for responding effectively.

- **Constructive Criticism**: This feedback is specific, actionable, and focused on behaviors or outcomes. For example, "Your presentation was engaging, but adding more visuals could make your points even clearer."

- **Destructive Criticism**: This type of feedback is vague, harsh, or aimed at personal attributes rather than actions. For instance, "Your presentation was boring and pointless" lacks actionable insights and serves only to demean.

Learning to recognize these distinctions allows you to focus on feedback that fosters growth and disregard what doesn't serve you.

Filtering Feedback Effectively

To make the most of feedback, apply the following strategies to filter and assess its value:

1. Assess the Intent: Determine whether the feedback is offered with the goal of helping you improve or simply to criticize. Constructive feedback is usually well-meaning and aimed at fostering growth.

2. Look for Specificity: Valuable feedback is detailed and actionable, offering clear guidance for improvement. If it's vague or overly critical, it may not warrant much attention.

3. Consider the Source: Is the feedback coming from someone who understands your work or has your best interests at heart? Feedback from a trusted and knowledgeable source carries more weight.

Distinguishing Constructive vs. Destructive Criticism

Not all criticism is created equal. Understanding the difference between constructive and destructive criticism is crucial for deciding how to respond.

- **Constructive Criticism**: This type of feedback is specific, actionable, and focused on behaviors or outcomes. For example, "Your presentation was engaging, but adding more visuals could make your points even clearer."

- **Destructive Criticism**: Often vague, overly harsh, or focused on personal attributes, this type of feedback aims to belittle. For instance, "Your presentation was boring and pointless" offers no actionable insights and serves only to demean.

How to Filter Feedback:

1. **Assess the Intent**: Ask yourself if the feedback is meant to help you improve or simply to criticize.

2. **Look for Specificity**: Constructive criticism is clear and actionable. If the feedback is vague, it may not be worth engaging with.

3. **Consider the Source**: Is the feedback coming from someone who understands your work or has your best interests at heart?

By distinguishing between the two, you can focus on constructive criticism that aids your development while letting go of destructive comments that serve no purpose.

Responding with Grace

Criticism, even when constructive, can trigger an emotional response. Responding with grace requires emotional regulation and a willingness to engage with feedback constructively.

Steps to Respond Gracefully:

1. **Pause and Breathe**: Before reacting, take a moment to process your emotions. This prevents defensive or impulsive responses.

2. **Express Gratitude**: Acknowledge the effort the other person took to provide feedback. For example, "Thank you for taking the time to share your thoughts."

3. **Ask Clarifying Questions**: Seek specific examples or suggestions. For instance, "Could you give me an example of what you mean by 'more engaging visuals'?"

4. **Reflect on the Feedback**: Take time to analyze the criticism objectively. Consider what resonates and how you can apply it.

Responding this way not only demonstrates maturity but also fosters an environment of mutual respect and continuous improvement.

Examples of Constructive Responses

Consider these scenarios to illustrate how to handle criticism with grace:

- **Scenario 1**: Your manager tells you that your team meetings lack focus.
  Response: "I appreciate the feedback. Can you share specific ways I could structure the meetings better?"

- **Scenario 2**: A peer comments that your email communication is too brief and lacks detail.
  Response: "Thank you for pointing that out. Could you let me know what specific information would make my emails clearer?"

These examples highlight the importance of curiosity and collaboration when addressing criticism.

Case Study: Rob's Presentation Skills

Rob, a junior analyst, struggled with public speaking. After a presentation, his supervisor commented, "Your analysis was thorough, but your delivery needs more energy to engage the audience." Initially, Rob felt embarrassed and frustrated, interpreting the comment as a critique of his personality.

After reflecting, Rob realized the feedback was about his presentation style, not his worth. He joined a local Toastmasters group to practice public speaking and sought advice from colleagues known for their engaging presentations. Over time, Rob's delivery improved dramatically, and he became a sought-after speaker in his company.

Interactive Exercises

1. Feedback Analysis Chart Create a chart to analyze recent feedback:

- **Column 1**: The feedback you received.
- **Column 2**: Was it constructive or destructive?
- **Column 3**: What can you learn from it?
- **Column 4**: Action steps to apply or dismiss the feedback.

2. Role-Playing Exercise Pair up with a friend or colleague and practice giving and receiving feedback. Take turns providing constructive criticism and responding to it gracefully. Reflect on what felt helpful and what could be improved in the exchange.

3. Criticism Journal Keep a journal to document feedback you've received:

- What was the feedback?
- How did it make you feel initially?
- What action did you take (or not take) as a result?
  Over time, this journal will help you track patterns in your responses and identify areas for growth.

Turning Feedback into Action

Criticism, when approached constructively, aids in personal and professional development. By reframing feedback, distinguishing between constructive and destructive criticism, and responding with grace, you turn critique into a tool for growth. As you practice these skills, you'll find that feedback, rather than being a source of anxiety, becomes an essential part of your journey to becoming your best self.

3.4 Turning Setbacks into Opportunities

Setbacks are inevitable, but how you perceive and respond to them determines their impact on your growth. While they may feel like failures in the moment, setbacks can be powerful catalysts for change and improvement when viewed through the right lens. This section explores how to adopt a growth mindset, extract valuable lessons from challenges, and regain confidence through small victories. By embracing setbacks as opportunities, you can foster resilience and uncover paths to success that might otherwise remain hidden.

The Growth Mindset

The idea of a growth mindset, pioneered by psychologist Carol Dweck, emphasizes the belief that skills and intelligence can be cultivated through persistence and effort. This mindset reframes failure as a catalyst to success rather than an insurmountable obstacle. For example, when Olivia, a small business owner, faced her first product launch flop, she initially felt defeated. However, instead of giving up, she analyzed customer feedback, improved her product, and ultimately created a best-seller. By focusing on what could be learned, Olivia turned her setback into a defining moment of growth.

How to Cultivate a Growth Mindset:

- **Reframe Failure:** Instead of saying, "I failed," try saying, "I learned what doesn't work."

- **Ask Constructive Questions:** Consider, "What can this teach me?" or "How can I improve next time?"

- **Adopt the Language of Progress:** Replace "I'm not good at this" with "I'm still learning how to do this."

Learning from Setbacks

Turning setbacks into opportunities begins with introspection. Conducting a personal SWOT (Strengths, Weaknesses, Opportunities, Threats) analysis is a practical way to evaluate what went wrong and why. For instance, let's revisit Olivia's product launch. Through her SWOT analysis, she identified:

- **Strengths:** Her product's unique features.

- **Weaknesses:** Poor market research.

- **Opportunities:** Engaging with a niche audience.

- **Threats:** Rising competition in her industry.

This structured reflection allowed her to develop an actionable plan for her next launch. She conducted thorough market research, connected with her target audience through social media, and created a tailored marketing campaign. The second launch succeeded, not despite the setback but because of it.

Interactive Exercise: Your Personal SWOT Analysis

1. **Choose a Recent Setback:** Reflect on a specific event or challenge.

2. **Complete Your SWOT Chart:** Divide a page into four sections—strengths, weaknesses, opportunities, and threats. List relevant points under each category.

3. **Develop an Action Plan:** Write down three steps to address your weaknesses and leverage your strengths.

This process not only helps you make sense of the setback but also equips you with strategies to move forward.

Celebrating Small Wins

Regaining confidence after a setback is a gradual process that begins with small, achievable goals. Each minor victory builds momentum, reminding you of your capabilities and fostering resilience. For example, when Andrew didn't secure a promotion he worked hard for, he was initially disheartened. Instead of dwelling on the disappointment, he set smaller goals: attending professional development workshops, networking with colleagues, and improving his leadership skills. Each step brought him closer to his ultimate goal while restoring his confidence.

Why Small Wins Matter:

- **They Build Momentum:** Small victories fuel motivation, making larger goals feel attainable.

- **They Reinforce Progress:** Focusing on what you've achieved reduces feelings of stagnation.

- **They Boost Resilience:** Success, even in small doses, reminds you of your ability to overcome challenges.

Ways to Celebrate Small Wins:

- Write down your achievements in a "success journal."

- Share your progress with a trusted friend or mentor.

- Reward yourself with something meaningful, like a favorite treat or a day off.

Real-Life Example: Bouncing Back from a Career Setback

Consider Maria, a marketing professional who lost her job during a company downsizing. Initially, she felt overwhelmed by rejection and uncertainty. However, Maria decided to view the situation as an opportunity to explore her interests. She took online courses in digital marketing, a field she had been curious about, and built a portfolio of freelance projects. By the time she was ready to re-enter the job market, Maria not only found a new role but also increased her salary and job satisfaction. Her setback became a launching pad for personal and professional growth.

Transforming Setbacks into Building Blocks

Setbacks don't have to define your story—they can enrich it. They encourage you to reassess, recalibrate, and reinvent yourself. By adopting a growth mindset, analyzing challenges constructively, and celebrating progress along the way, you can turn even the most difficult experiences into opportunities for growth. Each setback, when approached with resilience and determination, becomes a building block toward a stronger, more empowered version of yourself.

3.5 Emotional Balance in High-Pressure Situations

In today's fast-paced and demanding world, maintaining emotional balance under pressure is a crucial skill. It's not just about staying calm—it's about navigating challenging situations with clarity, composure, and confidence. Emotional balance allows you to make thoughtful decisions, communicate effectively, and remain adaptable even in the most high-stakes scenarios. This section explores practical techniques, strategies, and exercises to help you cultivate emotional balance and thrive under pressure.

Practical Techniques for Maintaining Composure

Deep Breathing:

When stress levels spike, your body's natural response is often shallow, rapid breathing, which can exacerbate anxiety. Deep breathing is a powerful tool to counteract this.

- **How to Practice**: Inhale deeply through your nose for a count of four, holding your breath for another four counts, and then slowly exhaling through your mouth for a count of six. Repeat for a few minutes until you feel more centered.

- **Case Example:** During a high-pressure sales pitch, Jake noticed his hands trembling and his thoughts racing. By practicing deep breathing for two minutes, he calmed his nerves and delivered his presentation with confidence.

Visualization:

Visualization involves mentally rehearsing success before entering a stressful situation.

- **How to Practice:** Close your eyes and picture yourself confidently and calmly handling the challenge. Imagine every detail—from your posture and tone of voice to the positive reactions of those around you.

- **Application:** A student about to take a major exam might visualize themselves calmly answering each question, reinforcing a sense of control and competence.

Time Management:

Feeling overwhelmed often stems from poor time management. Learning to prioritize tasks can prevent unnecessary stress.

- **How to Practice:** Create a daily schedule that separates tasks into urgent, important, and less critical categories. Focus on completing one priority at a time.

- **Interactive Activity:** Use a time-blocking worksheet to organize your day, allocating specific time slots for each priority.

Developing Emotional Intelligence

Emotional intelligence (EI) refers to the capacity to identify, comprehend, and regulate your own emotions while also understanding and empathizing with the emotions of others. In high-pressure situations, EI helps you regulate your reactions and maintain productive relationships.

Key Components of Emotional Intelligence:

1. **Self-Awareness:** Recognize your emotional triggers and how they influence your responses.

2. **Self-Regulation:** Practice managing your emotions rather than letting them control your actions.

3. **Empathy:** Understand and consider the perspectives of others, especially in tense interactions.

4. **Social Skills:** Communicate effectively, even in stressful circumstances, to foster collaboration and resolve conflicts.

Exercises for Emotional Balance

Empathy Walk:

- **Purpose:** Strengthen your ability to see situations from another's perspective.

- **How to Practice:** Choose a recent conflict or high-pressure moment. Reflect on how the other person might have felt and what pressures or motivations influenced their behavior. Write down your reflections and how you might approach a similar situation differently in the future.

Pause and Reframe:

- **Purpose:** Train yourself to respond rather than react.

- **How to Practice:** When faced with a stressful situation, take a moment to pause before speaking or acting. Ask yourself, "What is the best way to approach this that aligns with my goals and values?"

- **Example:** Instead of reacting angrily to a critical email, use this pause to draft a professional response that addresses the concerns raised constructively.

Body Scan Meditation:

- **Purpose:** Reduce physical tension caused by stress.

- **How to Practice:** Sit in a comfortable position and close your eyes. Slowly direct your attention to different parts of your body, starting at your toes and moving upward. Notice any areas of tension and imagine releasing that tension with each breath.

- **Application:** This exercise is particularly effective before high-pressure meetings or presentations.

Interactive Activity: Emotional Triggers Journal

1. **Track Stressful Moments:** Over the course of a week, note situations that caused stress or emotional imbalance.

2. **Identify Triggers:** Write down what triggered your emotions and how you initially responded.

3. **Reflect and Strategize:** For each trigger, brainstorm one or two alternative responses you could use next time to maintain emotional balance.

Building Resilience in High-Stakes Situations

Developing emotional balance doesn't happen overnight—it's a skill that requires practice and self-awareness. Each time you employ these techniques, you strengthen your ability to remain composed and effective under pressure. By integrating these practices into your daily life, you'll find that high-pressure situations become opportunities to demonstrate growth, confidence, and resilience.

Mastering Time Management

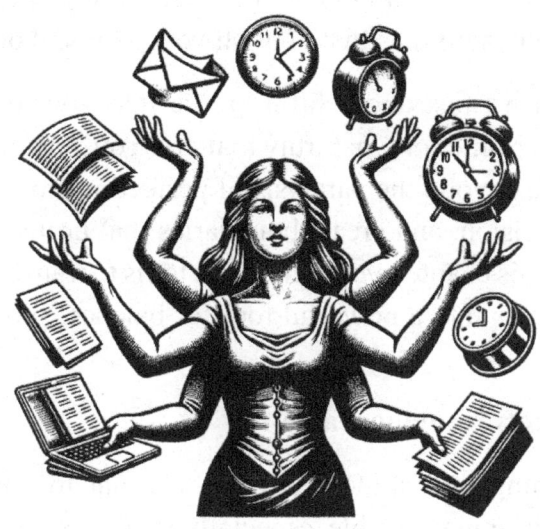

Picture this: your calendar is brimming with back-to-back appointments, unrelenting deadlines, and a seemingly endless list of reminders. You feel as if you're sprinting on a treadmill, constantly trying to catch up, but the finish line keeps moving farther away. Sound familiar? This relentless pace can feel suffocating, especially for perfectionists. The harder you try to optimize your time, the more elusive it becomes, leaving you overwhelmed and drained.

Why does this happen? Perfectionism often manifests as a desire to control every detail and ensure everything is done flawlessly. But this pursuit of perfection can backfire, creating inefficiencies and eating up precious time. Instead of getting ahead, you feel stuck in a cycle of over-analysis, procrastination, and mounting stress. Time, once your most valuable resource, starts to feel like your biggest enemy.

But what if you could rewrite this narrative? What if time could become your ally instead of your adversary? Imagine approaching each day with clarity, focus, and confidence, knowing that you're using your time in ways that align with your values and priorities. Picture having the freedom to not only meet your responsibilities but also to engage in activities that nourish your soul and bring you joy.

This chapter isn't just about fitting more into your day; it's about reclaiming your time for what truly matters. You'll learn strategies to help you move beyond the paralysis of perfectionism, prioritize your tasks with precision, and create boundaries that protect your energy. By the end of this chapter, you'll have the tools to transform time from a source of stress into a powerful tool for balance, productivity, and fulfillment.

Why Time Feels Unmanageable

Before launching into strategies, it's important to understand *why* time often feels unmanageable, especially for perfectionists. Consider the following common scenarios:

- **Overcommitment:** You say "yes" to everything, fearing that declining might disappoint others or reflect poorly on you. Over time, your plate becomes so full that even small tasks feel monumental.

- **Over-analysis:** Instead of making quick decisions, you agonize over every choice, afraid of making the wrong one. This not only wastes time but also drains your mental energy.

- **Avoidance of Imperfection:** Tasks that could be completed in an hour stretch into days because you keep revisiting them, searching for ways to make them better—even when "better" isn't necessary.

- **Lack of Prioritization:** With so much to do, you spend your time on urgent but unimportant tasks, leaving little room for what truly matters.

These habits are fueled by the fear of falling short, but the irony is that they often lead to falling behind. By recognizing these patterns, you can begin to dismantle them and build a healthier relationship with your time.

The Role of Mindset in Time Management

At the heart of effective time management lies a mindset shift. Instead of striving to do everything perfectly, aim to do the right things well. This doesn't mean settling for mediocrity—it means channeling your energy into what matters most.

The Myth of Multitasking

Many perfectionists pride themselves on being able to juggle multiple tasks at once, believing it makes them more efficient. However, research shows that multitasking often decreases productivity. When you split your focus, you're more likely to make mistakes and take longer to complete each task.

Reflection Prompt:

Think about a recent time when you multitasked. How did it affect the quality and timing of your work? What could you have done differently if you focused on one task at a time?

The Power of Progress

Progress, not perfection, is the key to effective time management. When you focus on making steady progress rather than achieving flawless results, you free yourself from the paralysis of overthinking.

Example: Instead of spending hours perfecting a presentation, aim to complete it to the best of your ability in a set amount of time. Then, use any remaining time for minor refinements, if necessary.

Reframing Failure

Fear of failure often drives perfectionism, leading to procrastination and inefficiency. Reframe failure as a learning opportunity rather than a reflection of your worth. Every mistake is a step closer to mastery.

Case Study:

Lindsey, a perfectionist graphic designer, used to spend days revising client drafts. She realized that her clients were more impressed by her ability to meet deadlines than by minor tweaks they rarely noticed. By embracing a mindset of "good enough," Lindsey not only saved time but also reduced her stress levels.

Setting the Stage for Success

Effective time management isn't just about strategies; it's also about creating the right environment for success.

1. **Declutter Your Space:** A cluttered workspace often leads to a cluttered mind. Take 10 minutes each day to organize your desk, digital files, or calendar. A clear space fosters a clear mind.

2. **Determine Your Most Productive Times:** Each person has specific periods during the day when their focus and energy levels are at their highest.

Interactive Exercise:

- For one week, track your energy levels and focus throughout the day.
- Note patterns and adjust your schedule accordingly.

3. **Eliminate Time Thieves**: Identify habits or activities that steal your time without adding value. Frequent distractions often stem from activities like excessive use of social media, attending unnecessary meetings, or repeatedly checking emails.

Challenge:

Commit to limiting one time-thieving activity this week. For instance, set a timer for social media use or designate specific times to check emails.

A Roadmap for Reclaiming Your Time

The journey to mastering time management isn't about squeezing every second out of your day—it's about using your time intentionally. Here's a roadmap to guide you:

1. **Reflect on Your Values:** What matters most to you? Align your schedule with your priorities.

2. **Embrace Flexibility:** Life is unpredictable. Allow room for adjustments without guilt.

3. **Celebrate Small Wins:** Each step toward reclaiming your time is a victory. Acknowledge your progress.

Interactive Exercise: Your Ideal Day

- Picture your perfect day from morning to evening. What activities would you choose to spend your time on?

- Compare this vision to your current schedule. Identify one change you can make this week to bring your reality closer to your ideal.

4.1 Time Management for Perfectionists

Perfectionism, while often praised as a trait of high achievers, can sabotage your ability to manage time effectively. Tasks that could take minutes balloon into hours as you agonize over every detail. This cycle of over-analysis leads to procrastination, stress, and missed opportunities, creating a spiral of inefficiency.

Case Study: Ameila's Report Dilemma

Ameila is a project manager known for her meticulous work ethic. When tasked with preparing a weekly progress report, she spent the entire weekend perfecting it. She agonized over the font size, debated word choices, and even triple-checked data that was already verified. Her family missed her presence at Sunday dinner, and she started Monday morning exhausted and behind on other tasks.

When she submitted the report, her boss skimmed it for two minutes, gave it a "great," and moved on.

The takeaway? The extra hours Amelia spent chasing perfection didn't add value. Instead, her time could have been better utilized balancing her priorities.

Actionable Strategies to Break the Cycle

When perfectionism takes hold, it often feels like there's no finish line. You may find yourself stuck in endless loops of revisions, rechecking, and hesitation, unable to declare a task complete. Breaking this cycle starts with rethinking your approach to success— not as flawless execution, but as meaningful progress. By shifting your mindset and adopting practical strategies, you can free yourself from the paralysis of perfectionism and make room for growth and achievement.

Adopt the "Good Enough" Mindset

Perfectionism thrives on the fear of falling short. Replacing this with a "good enough" mindset shifts your focus to progress and completion. This doesn't mean settling for mediocrity; rather, it's about recognizing when a task is complete and moving on.

- **The Pareto Principle (80/20 Rule):** Identify the 20% of tasks that yield 80% of the results. For example, instead of reworking every slide in a presentation, prioritize the most impactful visuals or talking points.

- **Mantra for Progress:** Repeat to yourself, "Done is better than perfect," whenever you feel stuck in a loop of over-analysis.

Interactive Activity: Done, Not Perfect

Objective: Reduce procrastination and celebrate progress.

1. **List three tasks you've been avoiding** because you feel they need to be "perfect." Examples might include replying to an email, organizing your workspace, or drafting a report.

2. **Set a timer** for each task (e.g., 20–30 minutes). Commit to completing the task within that timeframe, focusing on function over perfection.

3. **Evaluate your feelings:** After each task, take a moment to reflect. Did completing it feel satisfying? Did your "good enough" work meet the actual needs of the task?

4. **Celebrate Completion:** Reward yourself after finishing all three tasks, whether it's a short break, a favorite snack, or simply acknowledging your progress.

Time-Blocking for Focus and Efficiency

Time-blocking is a structured approach to managing your day, where you allocate specific time slots for tasks and activities. This technique helps you avoid perfectionist tendencies by imposing time constraints.

Example Daily Schedule:

- **9:00–10:30 AM:** Deep focus (e.g., writing, data analysis).
- **10:30–11:00 AM:** Break (walk, snack, or mindfulness exercise).
- **11:00–12:00 PM:** Respond to emails.
- **12:00–1:00 PM:** Lunch and recharge.
- **1:00–2:30 PM:** Collaborative tasks (e.g., team meetings or brainstorming).

Pro Tip: Use tools like Google Calendar, Microsoft To-Do, or a paper planner to block time. Include buffers for flexibility and unexpected interruptions.

Combatting Decision Fatigue

Decision fatigue occurs when you overanalyze or make too many decisions in a day, leaving you mentally exhausted. Simplifying decisions can conserve your energy for what truly matters.

Practical Strategies:

1. **Streamline Routines:**

   o Plan meals for the week to avoid daily meal-decision stress.

   o Simplify your wardrobe by creating a "capsule wardrobe" of interchangeable essentials.

2. **Use Decision Frameworks:** Evaluate tasks based on their:

   o **Priority**: Does this task need immediate attention?

   o **Impact**: Will this task significantly affect your goals?

   o **Alignment**: Does it reflect your core values?

3. **Automate Repetitive Decisions:** Use tools like auto-bill pay, recurring task reminders, or automated grocery deliveries to reduce the mental load.

4.2 Prioritizing What Truly Matters

Time is one of life's most precious and finite resources, and how you choose to spend it shapes the quality of your life. Yet, in the hustle and bustle of daily demands, it's easy to lose sight of what truly matters. Too often, we find ourselves saying "yes" to everything, only to feel overcommitted, stretched thin, and unfulfilled. Effective prioritization isn't about squeezing more into an already packed schedule—it's about cutting through the noise and intentionally directing your focus and energy toward what aligns with your deepest values and aspirations.

When you prioritize based on what you value most, every action takes on greater meaning. Instead of being driven by urgency or external pressures, you become guided by purpose and clarity. This approach not only reduces stress but also fosters a sense of fulfillment, joy, and long-term well-being. By aligning your actions with what you hold dear—whether it's family, personal growth, career success, or community contributions—you empower yourself to create a life that feels authentic and meaningful. In this section, we'll explore practical tools and strategies to help you identify, prioritize, and honor what truly matters, making each moment count.

Case Study: John's Overwhelmed To-Do List

John, a busy entrepreneur, found himself buried under an endless stream of tasks. From answering emails to attending back-to-back meetings, his days felt chaotic and unproductive. After learning about the Eisenhower Matrix, he categorized his tasks and discovered that many were urgent but not important. By delegating tasks like email responses and eliminating trivial activities, John freed up his schedule to focus on strategic planning and daily exercise—two priorities that aligned with his goals and values.

The result? Increased productivity, reduced stress, and a greater sense of purpose in his work.

Tools to Prioritize

Eisenhower Matrix

This simple but effective framework helps you sort tasks by urgency and importance:

- **Urgent & Important**: Handle these immediately (e.g., deadlines, emergencies).
- **Not Urgent but Important**: Schedule time to address these (e.g., long-term projects, personal development).

- **Urgent but Not Important**: Delegate these tasks (e.g., scheduling appointments).

- **Not Urgent & Not Important**: Eliminate them entirely (e.g., excessive scrolling on social media).

Interactive Activity: Declutter Your To-Do List

1. **Write Down Tasks**: List every task you plan to complete today.

2. **Sort Tasks into Quadrants**: Use the Eisenhower Matrix to categorize them.

3. **Take Action**: Commit to tackling one **Important & Not Urgent** task first.

4. **Reflect**: At the end of the day, evaluate how prioritizing affected your focus and productivity.

Value-Based Goal Setting

Your time should align with your personal values and long-term aspirations. By grounding your decisions in your values, you'll naturally prioritize what truly matters.

1. **Identify Core Values**: Think about what's most important to you—family, health, creativity, career, or community.

2. **Evaluate Your Schedule**: Look at your calendar for the week. Do your activities reflect these values?

3. **Adjust as Needed**: If you value health but never have time for exercise, schedule it as a non-negotiable part of your day.

Case Study: Maria's Family First Approach

Maria, a realtor and mother of two, found herself constantly working late, missing family dinners, and feeling disconnected from her children. After identifying her core values—family, personal growth, and career success—she adjusted her schedule. Maria started leaving work on time twice a week to enjoy family dinners and set aside

Sunday afternoons for self-care. By realigning her time with her values, Maria found greater satisfaction and balance.

Flexible Prioritization for Life's Changes

Life is unpredictable, and your priorities may shift with time. Flexible prioritization helps you adapt to new challenges and opportunities without losing focus on what's essential.

1. **Reassess Regularly**: Schedule quarterly check-ins to evaluate whether your current priorities still align with your goals and values.

2. **Be Open to Change**: Embrace new opportunities or let go of outdated commitments as your circumstances evolve.

3. **Celebrate Growth**: Recognize how adapting your priorities helps you grow and thrive.

Case Study: Kevin's Career Pivot

Kevin spent years prioritizing his career as a corporate lawyer, but after a health scare, he realized he had neglected his personal well-being. He decided to scale back his workload, prioritize exercise, and pursue his passion for photography on weekends. Kevin's shift in priorities led to improved health and a renewed sense of purpose.

By regularly reassessing your priorities and aligning them with what truly matters, you create a roadmap for a life filled with intention and fulfillment. Let this be the foundation for how you approach each day, week, and year ahead.

4.3 Setting Boundaries Without Guilt

Boundaries are vital for protecting your time, energy, and mental well-being. They are like fences around your most precious resources, ensuring they're not depleted by unnecessary demands or distractions. Setting boundaries is not about shutting people out—it's about ensuring that you have the bandwidth to focus on what truly matters to you, whether it's personal growth, meaningful relationships, or achieving professional goals.

However, many of us struggle with setting and enforcing boundaries, often due to feelings of guilt or fear of disappointing others. This section explores actionable strategies, real-life examples, and interactive exercises to help you create and maintain boundaries with confidence and compassion.

Why Boundaries Matter

When boundaries are unclear or nonexistent, you risk burnout, resentment, and a loss of control over your time. On the other hand, clear boundaries:

- Protect your priorities.
- Allow you to say "yes" to what aligns with your values.
- Reduce stress by creating structure in your life.

Case Study: Julie's Overcommitted Calendar:

Julie, a team lead at a marketing agency, often found herself staying late at work. She couldn't say no to last-minute tasks from her boss or requests for help from her team. This left her feeling exhausted and resentful. After taking a boundary-setting workshop, Sarah learned to say no gracefully and delegate tasks effectively.

When her boss asked her to take on another project, she replied, "I'm currently focused on two high-priority projects. I can take this on if we shift one of my existing responsibilities." Her boss appreciated her clarity, and Julie found she could leave work on time without guilt.

The lesson: Boundaries create respect, not resentment.

Strategies for Assertive Boundaries

Prepared Scripts:

Having ready-made responses for common boundary challenges can make saying no feel more natural.

- **Work Example:** "I'd love to help, but I'm at capacity right now. Can we revisit this next week?"

- **Personal Example:** "I need this evening for myself. Let's reschedule our catch-up for another time."

- **Family Example:** "I know this is important, but I've committed to another priority. Let's find another way to make this work."

Interactive Activity: Create Your Boundary Toolkit

1. Identify three situations where you often struggle to set boundaries (e.g., work, family, social events).

2. Write one prepared script for each situation.

3. Practice these scripts aloud to gain confidence.

Handling Pushback:

It's natural for others to challenge your boundaries, especially if they're used to having unlimited access to your time. Consistency is key when faced with pushback.

- **Example Response**: "I understand this is important to you, but I need to prioritize my current commitments. I'm happy to revisit this later."

- **Key Tip:** Use the "broken record" technique. Calmly and respectfully repeat your boundary as needed. For example:

  o Them: "But I really need this done now."

  o You: "I hear you, but I must focus on my current deadline. Let's discuss this tomorrow."

Interactive Exercises

1. Personal Boundary Statement Exercise: Write down one boundary you want to set this week. For example:

- "I will not check work emails after 6 PM."

- "I will decline invitations that interfere with my Sunday self-care routine."

Practice communicating this boundary with a trusted friend or in front of a mirror. Reflect on how it feels to assert your needs confidently.

2. Boundary Roll-Play: Pair up with a friend or colleague and role-play common scenarios where boundaries are tested. For instance:

- A coworker asks you to take on extra work.

- A family member interrupts your personal time.

- A friend pressures you to attend a social event you're not interested in.

Take turns practicing how to respond assertively, using prepared scripts and the broken record technique.

3. Boundary Success Journal: Keep a journal of your boundary-setting experiences over the next week. For each instance:

- Note the situation and how you responded.

- Reflect on how it felt to enforce your boundary.

- Identify any pushback and how you handled it.

Review your entries at the end of the week to celebrate your progress and identify areas for improvement.

Building Long-Term Boundary Habits

Establishing boundaries is a continuous process, not a one-time event. Over time, consistent boundary-setting teaches others to respect your limits and strengthens your confidence.

Tips for Reinforcement:

- Communicate your boundaries clearly and proactively.

- Revisit your boundaries regularly to ensure they still align with your needs.

- Seek support from mentors, friends, or therapists if you struggle with persistent guilt or resistance.

By learning to set and maintain boundaries without guilt, you create the space and energy to focus on what truly matters. Remember: boundaries are not barriers—they are bridges to a more intentional, fulfilling life.

4.4 Timing-Saving Techniques for Busy Lives

Reclaiming time is not about squeezing more into an already packed schedule—it's about finding smarter ways to accomplish what truly matters. Time-saving techniques can help you streamline repetitive tasks, reduce decision fatigue, and maximize your energy for activities that align with your values. In this section, we'll explore practical strategies, real-life examples, and interactive exercises to help you regain control of your time.

The Power of Automation

Automation is like having an invisible assistant that takes care of the small but necessary tasks in your life. By automating repetitive activities, you free up mental space for more meaningful pursuits.

- Examples of Automation in Action:
  - Use Todoist or Trello for task reminders and project organization.
  - Set up recurring bill payments through your banking app.
  - Use apps like Zapier or IFTTT to create custom workflows, such as automatically saving email attachments to a specific folder in your cloud storage.

- **Case Study**: Emily's Automated Morning Routine Emily, a small business owner, felt overwhelmed by daily tasks like responding to emails and updating her social media. She implemented automation tools to schedule posts, send invoices, and even sort her email inbox. Within a month, Emily found she had two extra hours each day to focus on strategic planning.

Interactive Activity: Identify Automation Opportunities

1. List three repetitive tasks you perform weekly (e.g., paying bills, scheduling posts, sorting emails).

2. Research one app or tool that could help automate each task.

3. Implement one automation this week and track how much time it saves.

Batch Processing for Efficiency

Batch processing is a productivity powerhouse. By grouping similar tasks together, you minimize the time lost to context-switching, allowing you to work more efficiently.

- Examples of Batch Processing:
    - Email Management: Designate specific times each day for checking and responding to emails rather than handling them sporadically.
    - Meal Prep: Cook meals in bulk on Sundays to save time during busy weekdays.
    - Errands: Combine trips to the grocery store, post office, and pharmacy into a single outing.
- **Case Study: Jeremy's Focused Work Blocks** Jeremy, a graphic designer, used to feel scattered, juggling emails, client meetings, and creative work throughout the day. By scheduling separate time blocks for communication,

brainstorming, and designing, he found his work quality improved and deadlines became easier to meet.

Interactive Exercise: Create a Batch Schedule

1. Identify a category of tasks you frequently perform (e.g., emails, household chores, client meetings).

2. Dedicate specific time blocks to these tasks during the week.

3. Reflect at the end of the week: Did batching tasks save time or reduce stress?

The Art of Delegation

Delegation is not about passing off work; it's about leveraging the strengths of others to achieve shared goals. By identifying tasks that can be handled by someone else, you can focus on higher-priority activities.

- **Examples of Delegation:**

    o **At Work:** Assign a team member to compile data for a report.

    o **At Home:** Use a grocery delivery service or assign household chores to family members.

    o **In Life:** Hire a virtual assistant for administrative tasks.

Interactive Activity: Build a Delegation Plan

1. Write down five tasks you regularly perform that someone else could manage.

2. Identify a person or resource (e.g., family member, team member, external service) to delegate each task.

3. Delegate one task this week and observe the impact on your schedule and stress levels.

Minimizing Distractions

Distractions are time thieves, pulling your focus away from what truly matters. Creating an environment that supports deep work is essential for productivity.

Strategies to Minimize Distractions:

- o Device-Free Hours: Schedule specific periods when you turn off notifications and avoid screens.

- o Headphones & Music: Use noise-canceling headphones or calming background music to block out external noise.

- o Workspace Design: Keep your workspace clutter-free and visually appealing to reduce mental distractions.

Case Study: David's Distraction-Free Mornings

David, a software developer, struggled to focus in a noisy home environment. He implemented device-free mornings and invested in a pair of noise-canceling headphones. These changes allowed him to complete more work in less time, freeing up his afternoons for family activities.

Interactive Exercise: Create a Distraction-Free Zone

1. Identify the biggest distractions in your environment (e.g., noise, phone notifications, clutter).

2. Choose one strategy to address each distraction (e.g., setting a "do not disturb" time, using headphones, decluttering your desk).

3. Test your new distraction-free zone for a week and note any changes in productivity.

Reclaiming time is about more than squeezing efficiency out of every moment—it's about creating space for what truly matters. By automating, batching, delegating, and reducing distractions, you can free yourself from unnecessary stress and focus on the activities that align with your values and bring you joy.

4.5 Reclaiming Time for Personal Fulfillment

Reclaiming time for personal fulfillment is not a luxury—it's a necessity for a balanced and meaningful life. Often, we get so caught up in responsibilities that we neglect the activities and moments that rejuvenate our spirit. Let's examine some ways to help you carve out time for self-care and joy, transforming your schedule into one that supports your well-being.

The Importance of Non-Negotiable Self-Care

Think of self-care as recharging your battery—it's what allows you to show up fully in all aspects of your life. Scheduling regular self-care is an act of prioritizing your well-being.

- **Examples of Non-Negotiable Self-Care Activities:**
    - Morning yoga or stretching to set a calm tone for the day.
    - Journaling for 10 minutes before bed to reflect and unwind.
    - Engaging in creative pursuits like painting, crafting, or baking to stimulate joy.

Case Study: Abby's "Me-Time Mondays"

Abby, a busy nurse, struggled to find time for herself. She started blocking out one hour every Monday evening for an activity she loved—gardening. After just a month, Abby noticed she felt more grounded and had more patience for her demanding job and family obligations.

Interactive Activity: Design Your Self-Care Calendar

1. Choose one day each week to dedicate at least 30 minutes to self-care.

2. Write down three self-care activities that resonate with you.

3. Add these activities to your calendar as non-negotiable appointments.

Mindful Time Tracking: Awareness is Key

Mindful time tracking helps you uncover where your time is going and how you can redirect it to align with your values and priorities.

- **Steps for Mindful Time Tracking:**

    1. For one day, log every activity and the time spent on it. Be honest—this isn't about judgment, but awareness.

    2. At the end of the day, review your log and identify patterns. Which activities felt meaningful? Which felt like time-wasters?

    3. Adjust your schedule by reducing or eliminating activities that don't serve your goals or well-being.

- **Case Study: Tom's "Unintentional Scrolling"**

    Tom, a marketing executive, found that he spent nearly two hours each evening scrolling through social media. After tracking his time for a week, he decided to limit his scrolling to 15 minutes and use the extra time to read books he'd been wanting to explore. This small change brought him more relaxation and satisfaction.

Interactive Exercise: Track and Reclaim Your Time

1. Download a time-tracking app or use a simple notebook to log your activities for one day.

2. Highlight 1-2 activities where time could be better spent.

3. Commit to replacing these activities with something meaningful, such as a hobby, exercise, or quality time with loved ones.

Embracing a "Time Abundance" Mindset

Many people operate under a "time scarcity" mindset, always feeling that there's never enough time. Shifting to a "time abundance" mindset allows you to focus on the quality of your experiences rather than the quantity of tasks you complete.

- **How to Cultivate Time Abundance:**
    - Practice gratitude for the time you do have. Acknowledge and celebrate moments of joy, peace, or connection.
    - Slow down and savor small, everyday experiences, like enjoying your morning coffee or watching a sunset.
    - Let go of the pressure to fill every moment with activity.

- **Case Study: Lila's Evening Gratitude Ritual**

    Lila, a mother of two, started a simple gratitude practice each night. She would write down one "time-rich" moment from her day, such as laughing with her kids or walking in the park. Over time, this practice helped her feel more content and less rushed.

Interactive Reflection: Gratitude for Time-Rich Moments

1. At the end of each day, jot down one moment when you felt at ease or joyful.

2. Reflect on how that moment made you feel and how you can create more of those experiences.

Making Room for Joy

Joyful activities are often the first to be sacrificed when life gets busy, but they are essential for a fulfilling life.

- **Examples of Joyful Activities:**
  - Joining a dance class or experimenting with a new recipe.
  - Exploring nature through hiking or gardening.
  - Spending quality time with loved ones or pets.

Interactive Exercise: Plan Your Joyful Moment

1. Think of one activity that brings you genuine joy but that you've been neglecting.
2. Schedule this activity within the next week.
3. Share your plan with a friend or loved one to hold yourself accountable.

By prioritizing self-care, tracking how you spend your time, adopting a time abundance mindset, and building a balanced schedule, you can reclaim your time for personal fulfillment. These strategies aren't just about managing time—they're about honoring your needs, values, and joy. Embrace this approach to create a life that feels both meaningful and abundant.

Overcoming Fear of Failure

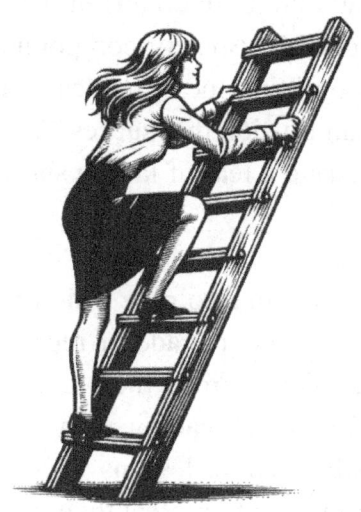

Consider standing on the edge of a diving board, toes gripping the edge, heart pounding. Below, the water looks inviting, but a small voice whispers, "What if I fail?" This hesitation, fueled by fear of imperfection, keeps many from taking the leap into new opportunities. Fear of failure isn't inherently negative—it's rooted in a natural desire to protect ourselves—but it often becomes a barrier to growth. To alleviate it, we need to review its origins and impact on our lives.

5.1 Understanding Fear of Failure

The Origins of Fear

Fear of failure often stems from a combination of cultural narratives, personal experiences, and biological instincts. These elements intertwine, shaping how we perceive risks and respond to challenges.

Cultural Expectations and Self-Worth

From a young age, many are taught to equate achievements with value. Comments like, "You're so smart for getting an A," while intended as praise, can subtly suggest that worth is tied to success. This mindset can grow into an internalized belief that anything less than perfect is unacceptable. Society compounds this by glorifying success stories, often omitting the struggles and failures that paved the way. This creates an illusion that success is linear and failure is a sign of weakness, fostering a fear of falling short.

Childhood Conditioning

Experiences in childhood can also play a significant role. Imagine a child who is scolded for a poor grade or receives praise only when they excel in sports. Over time, they may associate love and acceptance with performance, leading to an aversion to situations where failure is possible. These lessons become ingrained, and as adults, they might avoid risks to protect their sense of worth.

Biological Roots:

From an evolutionary perspective, fear exists as a survival mechanism. Our ancestors relied on fear to avoid threats, ensuring their safety. While this instinct once served to protect against physical harm, it now manifests in emotional and social contexts. Modern fears, such as public embarrassment or professional setbacks, trigger the same fight-or-flight response, often making challenges feel disproportionately daunting.

How Fear Influences Behavior

Fear of failure doesn't just affect emotions; it shapes decision-making and actions, often in subtle but significant ways.

- **Avoidance Behaviors**: Many perfectionists avoid situations where they might fail, opting for the safety of familiarity.

While this reduces immediate discomfort, it limits opportunities for growth and learning.

- **Over-Preparation**: To counteract fear, individuals might over-prepare, spending excessive time and energy on tasks to ensure success. This can lead to burnout and diminish productivity.

- **Procrastination**: Paradoxically, fear of failure often results in procrastination. The anxiety of starting a task where failure feels possible can lead to delays, reinforcing the fear in a cycle of inaction.

Case Study: Ava's Start-Up Stall

Ava dreamed of opening her bakery. However, the thought of failure paralyzed her. She told herself she needed more experience, more savings, and more planning. Years passed, and her dream remained just that—a dream. Looking back, Ava realized that fear, not external obstacles, had held her back.

The Takeaway: Fear of failure often costs more than failure itself. The real regret comes not from trying and falling short, but from never trying at all.

Interactive Exercise: Fear Audit

Confronting fear starts with understanding its roots. Use this exercise to identify and challenge your fear of failure:

1. **Identify a Goal or Opportunity You've Avoided**
   - Write down one thing you've been putting off due to fear.

2. **Name Your Fears**
   - Be specific. What scares you about this opportunity? *Examples*: "I'll embarrass myself," or "People will think I'm incompetent."

3. **Explore the Worst-Case Scenario**

   o Imagine the worst possible outcome. Write it down in detail.

   o Ask yourself:

      ▪ *How likely is this to happen?*

      ▪ *If it did, how would I recover?*

4. **Reframe the Fear**

   o What's the best-case scenario?

   o What's a realistic middle-ground outcome?

   o Recognize that the worst-case scenario is often far less catastrophic than imagined.

Reflection Prompt

What might you gain if you faced this fear? Write a few sentences about how this opportunity aligns with your values or goals.

Shifting Perspective: Failure as Feedback

One of the most transformative ways to reduce fear is to view failure as an opportunity for learning rather than a judgment of worth. Each misstep provides valuable insights that guide future success. Think of failure as a trusted teacher—it's not the end of the road but a necessary part of the journey.

Example

Imagine a scientist conducting experiments. They don't label failed experiments as personal failures; instead, they see them as data points leading to the next breakthrough. Adopting this mindset in daily life allows you to embrace challenges with curiosity rather than dread.

Interactive Activity: The "Failure as Feedback" Journal

1. Reflect on a recent mistake or perceived failure.

2. Answer the following prompts:

   o What did I learn from this experience?

   o What could I do differently next time?

   o How has this experience helped me grow?

This journaling exercise helps shift your mindset, encouraging you to view setbacks as growth points to success.

The Cycle of Fear and Perfectionism

Fear of failure often feeds perfectionism, creating a vicious cycle. The higher the standards you set, the greater the fear of falling short, which, in turn, fuels more perfectionist behaviors. Breaking this cycle requires awareness and intentional effort.

Visualization Technique:

Picture your fear as a large, closed door. On the other side of the door lies your goal. Instead of focusing on the size of the door, visualize yourself turning the handle and stepping through. Imagine how it feels to be on the other side, having faced and manage your fear.

Reflection Prompt:

What is one "door" you've avoided opening? What opportunities or possibilities lie beyond this challenge?

By exploring the roots of fear, identifying its influence, and reframing it as a learning opportunity, you take the first steps toward freedom from its grip.

5.2 Strategies for Facing Fear Head On

Facing fear can feel like standing in front of an insurmountable wall—daunting and immobilizing. Yet, courage isn't a trait reserved for the fearless; it's a skill cultivated through deliberate, incremental action. Fear thrives in the shadows of uncertainty and avoidance, often growing larger the longer it's left unchallenged. However, just as darkness recedes when a light is shone, fear diminishes when met with intention and action.

The key to overcoming fear isn't about leaping into the unknown all at once—it's about taking small, manageable steps that build confidence and resilience. Each step, no matter how small, acts as a victory, chipping away at fear's hold and creating a path forward. By confronting fear with thoughtful strategies, you can transform it from a paralyzing force into a motivator for growth and change.

This section offers practical tools and techniques to help you face fear head-on. These strategies are designed to empower you, helping you move through fear with intention, build self-assurance, and ultimately embrace challenges as opportunities for transformation. Whether your fear stems from public speaking, career changes, or personal vulnerabilities, these methods provide a roadmap to confront and manager the barriers holding you back.

Gradual Exposure

Fear often looms larger than reality. Gradual exposure involves breaking intimidating challenges into smaller, manageable steps, allowing you to face them incrementally and build confidence along the way.

Example

Imagine you're nervous about networking at professional events. Instead of plunging into a large conference, begin by initiating one-on-one conversations with coworkers or attending small-scale events. With each interaction, you develop the skills and courage needed for larger gatherings.

Case Study: Drew and Public Speaking

Drew was paralyzed by the thought of public speaking. To reduce his fear, he started small:

1. Practice: He rehearsed in front of a mirror to get comfortable with his material.

2. Feedback: He recorded himself and asked trusted friends for constructive feedback.

3. Progression: Drew began sharing ideas during team meetings and gradually moved to presenting at departmental gatherings.

Over several months, Drew transformed his fear into confidence, delivering a successful keynote speech at a company event.

Interactive Activity: Fear Hierarchy

Fear can feel insurmountable when viewed as a single challenge. Break it into smaller steps with this exercise:

1. **Identify Your Fear:** Choose a fear you want to overcome (e.g., public speaking, networking, or asking for a promotion).

2. **Create a Ladder:**

   o Step 1: Start small (e.g., practice in private or with close friends).

   o Step 2: Add moderate exposure (e.g., speak up in a meeting or attend a small event).

   o Step 3: Take on a bigger challenge (e.g., present at a team meeting or attend a larger event).

3. **Celebrate Progress**: Acknowledge each step completed as a victory, reinforcing your confidence.

Visualization Techniques

Visualization is a powerful tool for reducing fear and preparing for success. By mentally rehearsing a positive outcome, you condition your mind to approach challenges with optimism and readiness.

Exercise: The Power of Mental Rehearsal

1. Close your eyes and imagine a specific fear-inducing situation (e.g., delivering a presentation).

2. Picture every detail: the room, the audience, your tone of voice, and your body language.

3. Visualize yourself navigating the scenario with confidence, concluding with a successful outcome.

4. Repeat daily to reinforce this positive mental blueprint.

Why It Works: Visualization familiarizes your mind with the experience, reducing the "unknown" factor that amplifies fear. This repeated mental rehearsal helps you feel more prepared and capable when the time comes.

Cognitive Restructuring

Fear is often fueled by catastrophic thinking—assuming the worst-case scenario will occur. Cognitive restructuring helps you identify, challenge, and replace irrational fears with balanced perspectives.

Example

- Fear: "If I mess up this report, I'll lose my job."

- Challenge: "Has anyone ever lost their job over one mistake? Is this fear based on evidence or emotion?"

- Reframe: "Mistakes are learning opportunities. I'll do my best and address any feedback."

Interactive Activity: Thought Journal

Use this structured journaling exercise to address fear-based thoughts:

1. **Write Down the Thought**: Note when a fearful thought arises.

   o Example: "I'll embarrass myself in the meeting."

2. **Examine the Evidence**:

   o Supporting Evidence: "I feel nervous about speaking."

   o Contradicting Evidence: "I've spoken in meetings before and received positive feedback."

3. **Reframe the Thought**:

   o Balanced Perspective: "I may feel nervous, but I'm prepared and capable."

Review your thought journal regularly to identify patterns and track your progress in challenging negative thoughts.

Building a Fear-Handling Toolkit

Facing fear requires a set of tools to calm your mind and guide your actions. Here are some strategies to add to your toolkit:

1. **Progressive Muscle Relaxation**

   o Method: Systematically tense and relax each muscle group, starting from your toes and working upward.

   o Purpose: Reduces physical tension caused by fear, fostering a sense of calm.

2. **Mindful Breathing**

   o Method: Inhale deeply for a count of four, hold for four, and exhale for six.

   o Purpose: Slows your heart rate and quiets racing thoughts, bringing clarity and focus.

3. **Anchor Statements**

   o Create phrases that ground you in the moment, such as:

     - "I am capable and prepared."

     - "I've faced challenges before, and I can handle this."

   o Use these affirmations as reminders of your strength when fear strikes.

Case Study: Mia's Career Leap

Mia wanted to switch careers but was paralyzed by fear. She worried about leaving a stable job and failing in a new field. To manage her fear, Mia:

1. **Created a Fear Hierarchy**:

   o Step 1: Research new fields of interest.

   o Step 2: Network with professionals in those fields.

   o Step 3: Enroll in online courses to build relevant skills.

2. **Used Visualization**: Mia imagined herself succeeding in her new role, envisioning the fulfillment it would bring.

3. **Challenged Negative Thoughts**:

   o Fear: "I'll fail and regret leaving my current job."

   o Reframe: "This is a learning opportunity. Even if I face challenges, I'll gain valuable experience."

Six months later, Mia successfully transitioned to her new career, crediting her gradual, deliberate approach.

Interactive Exercise: Action Plan for Facing Fear

Use this activity to create a personalized plan for confronting one of your fears:

1. **Name the Fear**: What are you afraid of?

2. **Break It Down**: What smaller steps can you take to confront this fear?

3. **Visualize Success**: Imagine overcoming the fear. How will it feel?

4. **Set a Timeline**: When will you take the first step? The second?

5. **Reflect and Adjust**: After each step, reflect on what you've learned and adjust your plan if needed.

The Takeaway

Fear is a natural response, but it doesn't have to control you. By using strategies like gradual exposure, visualization, and cognitive restructuring, you can face your fears with confidence. Remember, every small step forward is a victory that brings you closer to your goals. As you practice these techniques, fear transforms from an obstacle into a stepping-stone for growth.

5.3 Reframing Failure for Growth

Failure often feels like the end of the road, a stark reminder of our imperfections. However, it's better understood as a building block— a necessary part of the journey toward growth and success. Failure provides valuable insights, revealing gaps, sharpening strategies, and fostering resilience. When we shift our perspective and embrace failure as an opportunity for feedback, we transform it into a powerful tool for personal and professional development.

Failure as Feedback

Viewing failure as a learning experience instead of a setback is key to reframing it positively. Every mistake or misstep highlights areas for improvement and offers lessons that success alone cannot teach.

These lessons can inform better decisions, refine approaches, and ultimately lead to stronger outcomes.

Case Study: Meaghan's Set-Up Struggles

Meaghan launched her first business with high hopes but underestimated the demand for her product. Her initial venture failed within a year, leaving her disheartened. However, instead of giving up, Meaghan analyzed her mistakes—poor market research and inadequate customer feedback—and applied those lessons to her next business. Armed with deeper insights, her second startup flourished, demonstrating the value of learning through failure.

Interactive Exercise: Reframe a Recent Failure

1. **Write About It**: Describe a recent failure in detail—what happened, why it occurred, and how you felt.

2. **Reflect on Lessons**: What did this experience teach you? Consider new skills, insights, or perspectives gained.

3. **Identify Growth**: Write down one specific way you've grown because of this failure, such as improved problem-solving. This exercise encourages a mindset shift, helping you see failure as a foundation for growth rather than a source of shame.

Flexible Goal-Setting

One way to neutralize the fear of failure is to set goals that emphasize learning and adaptability. Using the SMART framework (Specific, Measurable, Achievable, Relevant, Time-bound) helps structure goals, but incorporating flexibility acknowledges that setbacks are part of the process. Flexible goals focus on progress and improvement rather than perfection, reducing the anxiety associated with potential missteps.

Activity: Create a "Growth Goal"

1. Choose a goal that involves stepping outside your comfort zone, such as learning a new skill or tackling a challenging project.

2. Define success beyond the outcome—what will you learn, regardless of the result?

3. Set flexible timelines that allow for adjustments and unforeseen challenges. This approach shifts your focus from avoiding failure to embracing the process of learning and growth.

The Value of Resilience

Failures often build resilience, which is essential for long-term success. The ability to bounce back from setbacks strengthens your mental toughness and equips you to handle future challenges with greater confidence.

Case Study: Michael Jordan's Missed Shots

Michael Jordan, one of basketball's greatest players, missed over 9,000 shots during his career. Reflecting on these missed opportunities, he stated, "I've failed over and over and over again in my life. And that is why I succeed." His willingness to embrace failure as part of the journey underscores how resilience drives excellence.

Mindset Shifts: From Failure to Opportunity

Changing how you perceive failure involves more than logic—it requires emotional rewiring. By viewing setbacks as opportunities for innovation and creativity, you open yourself up to new possibilities.

Interactive Activity: Failure Reframe Journal

- Keep a journal where you record failures or setbacks.

- For each entry, write three positive outcomes or lessons learned.

- Reflect on how these experiences have shaped your personal or professional growth. Over time, this habit fosters a mindset that views failure as a progress marker rather than a roadblock.

Celebrating Failure

Rather than hiding failures, acknowledge and celebrate them as signs of effort and progress. This doesn't mean glorifying mistakes but recognizing the courage it takes to try and the growth that results from the attempt.

Activity: Failure Celebration

1. Identify a past failure you now see as a turning point.

2. Write a note of appreciation to yourself for taking the risk, highlighting how it contributed to your growth.

3. Share the story with a trusted friend or mentor to normalize conversations about failure.

By reframing failure as growth, you unlock its potential to teach, transform, and empower. When you view setbacks as part of the journey rather than the end, you free yourself to take risks, explore new opportunities, and realize your fullest potential.

Embracing Failure as a Tool for Innovation

Failure is a cornerstone of creativity and innovation. The world's greatest inventors, entrepreneurs, and leaders often credit their failures as the catalyst for their breakthroughs.

Case Study: Dyson's 5,127 Prototypes

James Dyson created 5,127 prototypes before perfecting his revolutionary vacuum cleaner. Each failed attempt revealed a new insight, bringing him closer to success. Today, his story underscores the idea that every failure is a step toward innovation.

The lesson: Every failed attempt provides information that sharpens your approach.

Interactive Activity: Failure Reframing Wheel

Create a "Failure Reframing Wheel" to visualize failure as part of growth:

1. Draw a circle and divide it into four quadrants labeled:

    o   What went wrong

    o   Lessons learned

    o   How I'll apply these lessons

    o   New opportunities arising from this failure

2. Use the wheel to process past failures or any future challenges.

This activity encourages a structured, reflective approach to failure, helping you see its value in your personal and professional life.

Building a "Failure Resilience Toolkit"

To transform failure into growth, equip yourself with tools and habits that foster resilience:

1. **Reflective Journaling**: Dedicate time each week to write about challenges and what you've learned from them.

2. **Failure Role Models**: Research stories of individuals who turned failure into success, such as Oprah Winfrey, Steve Jobs, or Serena Williams. Use their journeys as inspiration.

3. **Mantras for Growth**: Create affirmations to reframe failure, such as:

    o   "Failure is a temporary detour, not a permanent dead end."

o "Every misstep brings me closer to clarity."

Group Activity: The "Failure Exchange"

Gather with friends or colleagues and share a story of a recent failure. Each person offers insights on what they learned and how they've grown. Listening to others' stories helps normalize failure and highlights its universal role in success.

Final Reflection: Gratitude for Failure

Take a moment to reflect on how failure has shaped your journey:

- What failure taught you your greatest lesson?

- How did it redirect you to something better?

- How can you embrace failure more willingly in the future?

By consistently reframing failure as growth, you cultivate a mindset that thrives on learning, adapts to challenges, and welcomes opportunities. Through this practice, you transform failure from an obstacle into a powerful ally on your path to success.

5.4 Building Confidence Through Small Wins

Big wins are built on the foundation of small victories. When you focus on incremental achievements, you not only build momentum but also reinforce a belief in your abilities. Small wins might seem insignificant at first, but they create a ripple effect, leading to larger successes over time.

The Power of Small Steps

Small steps break overwhelming goals into manageable actions. Each small step completed is a success in its own right, affirming that progress is possible. This approach is particularly helpful for perfectionists, who may feel paralyzed by the weight of a daunting objective.

Case Study: Katy's Fitness Journey

Katy dreamed of running a marathon, but the thought of running 26.2 miles felt impossible. Instead of focusing on the end goal, she decided to take a small step forward. She began with a simple commitment: a 10-minute jog each morning. After two weeks, she felt confident enough to increase her jogs by five minutes. As her stamina grew, she signed up for a local 5K. Crossing the finish line at her first race gave her the boost she needed to continue training. Over the next year, Katy tackled a 10K, then a half marathon, and finally achieved her dream of completing a full marathon.

Takeaway: Incremental progress leads to transformational results. Each small success builds your confidence and propels you toward your larger goals.

Interactive Exercise: Daily Wins Journal

Objective: Cultivate a habit of recognizing and celebrating small victories.

Instructions:

1. At the end of each day, write down one accomplishment, no matter how minor.

    o Examples: "I sent an email I was procrastinating on," or "I took a 10-minute walk."

2. Review your entries weekly to see how far you've come.

3. Reflect on patterns: Which types of wins make you feel most proud or motivated?

Purpose: Over time, this exercise will serve as a tangible reminder of your progress, building self-esteem and encouraging you to keep moving forward.

Visualization for Confidence

Visualization is a powerful tool for building self-assurance. By mentally rehearsing success, you create a blueprint for real-world action.

Exercise: Success Scenario

1. Find a quiet place and close your eyes.
2. Picture yourself completing a challenging task successfully.
   - For example: delivering a presentation, running a race, or learning a new skill.
3. Focus on the sensory details: What do you see, hear, and feel? Imagine the pride and satisfaction of achieving your goal.
4. Repeat this visualization daily to reinforce confidence in your abilities.

Why It Works: Visualizing success reduces anxiety and prepares your mind to approach challenges with calm determination. It helps you "practice" success, even before taking the first step.

Reward Progress

Rewards reinforce positive behaviors and provide motivation to keep going. They act as milestones that celebrate the journey, not just the destination.

Examples of Reward Systems:

- **Short-Term Rewards**: Treat yourself to a favorite snack, a relaxing bath, or 30 minutes of guilt-free screen time after completing a small task.
- **Mid-Term Rewards**: After reaching a milestone, plan a small outing, buy a book you've wanted, or enjoy a movie night.

- **Long-Term Rewards**: Celebrate major achievements with a larger reward, such as a weekend trip, a special purchase, or a dinner with friends.

Building Confidence Through Community

Sharing your small victories with others creates accountability and builds a support network. Whether it's a friend, mentor, or online community, sharing progress invites encouragement and provides an extra layer of motivation.

Interactive Activity: Weekly Wins Circle

- **Find a group of peers** who are working toward similar goals.

- **Share one win each week** and offer encouragement to others.

- **Reflect on shared challenges** and brainstorm solutions as a team.

Benefit: Celebrating together fosters a sense of community and reinforces the importance of consistent effort.

5.5 Sustaining Momentum Despite Setbacks

Setbacks are an unavoidable part of life, but they don't have to signal the end of your journey. How you respond to setbacks defines your trajectory, turning potential roadblocks into stepping stones for growth. Sustaining momentum requires resilience, a strategic mindset, and the ability to draw strength from your support network. This section provides actionable strategies to help you recover from challenges and keep moving toward your goals.

Create a Setback Recovery Plan

When setbacks occur, they can feel overwhelming, but a structured approach helps you regain focus and direction.

Steps to Create Your Recovery Plan:

1. **Assess What Went Wrong**: Take time to objectively evaluate the situation. What elements or circumstances led to the setback? Was it due to circumstances outside your control, a lack of preparation, or unrealistic expectations?

2. **Identify Lessons Learned**: Consider the lessons you gained from the experience. Did it reveal skills to improve or areas to strengthen?

3. **Create Actionable Next Steps**: Develop a clear plan for moving forward. Focus on small, achievable actions that build momentum.

Case Study: Lily's Career Setback

Lily didn't get the promotion she had been eyeing for months. Initially disheartened, she chose to seek feedback from her supervisor. She discovered areas for growth and enrolled in a professional development course to enhance her leadership skills. Six months later, she reapplied and secured the promotion. The experience not only strengthened her abilities but also boosted her confidence in navigating challenges.

Interactive Activity: "What's Next?" Plan

Instructions:

1. Reflect on a recent setback in your life.

2. Answer these prompts:

   o What specific events led to the setback?

   o What lessons can you draw from the experience?

   o What are three actionable steps you can take to move forward?

3. Write your responses in a journal or worksheet and review them periodically.

This activity helps you shift focus from the setback itself to the opportunities it creates for learning and growth.

Lean on Support Networks

Sharing your struggles with trusted individuals can provide both motivation and perspective. A solid support network can also hold you accountable, helping you stay committed to your goals.

Strategies for Building and Utilizing a Support Network:

- **Identify Key Supporters**: List trusted friends, family members, mentors, or colleagues who can offer guidance and encouragement.

- **Share Your Goals**: Open up about your challenges and aspirations. Inviting others into your journey fosters connection and accountability.

- **Ask for Specific Feedback**: Whether it's advice on a project or emotional support, clear communication ensures you get the help you need.

Case Study: Jared's Support Circle

After losing a major client, Jared felt his confidence falter. He turned to his mentor and peers for advice. Their reassurance and practical suggestions helped him rebuild his business strategy, eventually securing new clients. Jared credits his support network for reigniting his motivation during a challenging period.

Progress Reviews: Celebrating Wins and Adjusting Goals

Momentum requires regular reflection on what's working and what isn't. Set aside time to review your goals, celebrate achievements, and identify areas needing adjustment.

Steps for a Progress Review:

1. **Evaluate Successes**: Write down recent achievements, no matter how small. Celebrate them as evidence of your progress.

2. **Identify Obstacles**: Reflect on any challenges or setbacks. What patterns are emerging, and how can you address them?

3. **Adjust Goals**: Ensure your goals remain realistic and aligned with your evolving priorities. Flexibility is key to maintaining momentum.

Example:

If your goal was to exercise five days a week but you've only managed three, adjust your goal to three and gradually increase it over time. Small victories build consistency and confidence.

Persistence Through Setbacks

Persistence is about showing up, even when it feels difficult. It's not just about powering through but adapting your approach to meet challenges head-on.

Case Study: Jill's Fitness Journey

Jill set a goal to run a marathon but sprained her ankle during training. Instead of giving up, she switched to swimming to maintain her fitness while recovering. Her persistence paid off, and she crossed the marathon finish line a year later.

Tips for Building Persistence:

- **Break Goals into Milestones**: Focusing on small steps makes big goals less daunting.

- **Remember Your "Why"**: Reflect on the deeper purpose behind your goals.

- **Celebrate Resilience**: Acknowledge your ability to adapt and persevere.

Final Reflection: The Power of Setbacks

Setbacks aren't the end—they're part of the process. Each challenge faced and managed builds strength and character. By developing a recovery plan, leaning on support, and embracing flexibility, you can transform obstacles into opportunities for growth.

Interactive Activity: Gratitude for Growth

1. Write down one setback you've faced this year.

2. List three positive outcomes or lessons from that experience.

3. Reflect on how it has shaped your personal growth.

This exercise fosters gratitude for the challenges that have propelled you forward, reinforcing a mindset that welcomes resilience and adaptability.

By applying these strategies, you'll not only sustain momentum but also build the confidence and resilience needed to thrive through life's ups and downs.

You're Halfway Through! Let's Celebrate Your Progress Together

You've made it halfway through *The Perfectionism Detox Workbook*! That's no small feat, and I hope you've found the tools and insights so far to be valuable on your journey toward a life of progress, not perfection.

As you've worked through these chapters, you've already taken meaningful steps toward redefining success, embracing self-compassion, and creating space for what truly matters. You've shown incredible dedication—and that's worth celebrating.

Now, I'd love to ask for your help in sharing this message with others. If this workbook has inspired you, encouraged you, or helped you see perfectionism in a new light, would you consider leaving a review?

Why Your Review Matters

Your review isn't just feedback—it's a way to help others discover the same value you've experienced. Whether it's a few words about a favorite strategy or a reflection on how this book is helping you shift your mindset, your voice could be the encouragement someone else needs to begin their journey.

When you share your thoughts:

- You guide others. Reviews help others decide if this book is right for them.
- You inspire change. Your story might resonate with someone struggling with perfectionism.
- You support this work. Honest reviews help spread the word so more people can benefit from these tools.

How to Leave a Review in Three Simple Steps

Leaving a review is quick and easy! Here's how you can do it:

1. **Visit the book's page**. Head to the retailer where you purchased *The Perfectionism Detox Workbook* (like Amazon, IngramSpark, or another platform).

2. Click **"Write a Customer Review"**. On the book's product page, scroll down to the review section. Look for a button or link that says "Write a Customer Review".

3. **Share Your Experience**. Write a few sentences about your favorite parts of the book, what you've learned so far, or how it's helped you. No need for perfection here (how fitting, right?). Short and sincere is always impactful!

Need Inspiration?

Here are a few ideas to get started:

- What's been your biggest takeaway so far?
- Was there a strategy, exercise, or section that really resonated with you?
- How has this workbook made a difference in your daily life?

✿ ✿ ✿ ✿ ✿ "The insights on mindfulness and letting go of the perfectionism trap were eye-opening. Highly recommend to anyone looking to make real, sustainable changes!"

A Heartfelt Thank You

Thank you for taking this journey with me. Your willingness to dive into these pages, reflect, and grow means so much. Whether or not you leave a review, please know how proud I am of the progress you've made so far.

Let's keep moving forward together—you're doing incredible work!

With Gratitude,

Stacey Bottone, Author of *Perfectionism Detox Workbook*

Delegation and Trust

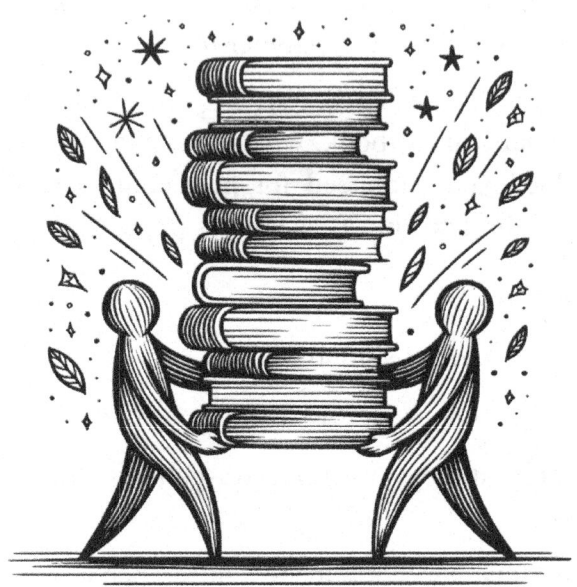

Envision standing in a bustling kitchen, where a chef orchestrates a culinary masterpiece. Every dish must be perfect, but it's not solely the chef's hands that bring the menu to life. It's the entire team—each member executing their part with precision. This scene mirrors the art of delegation, a vital skill in both personal and professional realms. Delegation is like conducting an orchestra, where each instrument plays its part to create a harmonious symphony.

Yet, for many of us, delegation feels like relinquishing control, inviting anxiety about whether tasks will be completed "just right." This hesitation often stems from the deeply ingrained belief that only *we* can ensure success. But holding onto every task, no matter how small, can lead to burnout, missed opportunities, and a sense of overwhelm. The truth is, effective delegation isn't about losing control—it's about empowering others while reclaiming your time and focus.

Mastering delegation has the power to transform not just your workload, but your mindset. By entrusting others with meaningful responsibilities, you create space to prioritize what truly matters— whether it's advancing your career, nurturing personal relationships, or investing in self-care. At the same time, you foster growth in those around you, giving them the opportunity to learn, contribute, and shine.

In this chapter, we'll explore why delegation is a cornerstone of effective time management and how to approach it with confidence and trust. You'll learn practical strategies to identify tasks that can— and should—be delegated, and how to overcome common barriers like fear of letting go or doubt in others' abilities. Together, we'll uncover how mastering delegation can lead to a more balanced, productive, and fulfilling life. Let's discover how sharing the load can empower you—and those around you—to achieve more.

6.1 The Power of Effective Delegation

Effective delegation is more than just assigning tasks; it's about creating a symbiotic relationship where responsibilities are shared, strengths are maximized, and growth is fostered on all sides. Delegation is the art of working smarter, not harder, and it empowers both the delegator and the team to reach new heights of productivity and fulfillment.

Case Study: Emily's Workload Overload

Emily, a marketing manager, was at her wit's end. Her daily to-do list felt never-ending, filled with meetings, emails, and tasks that left no room for strategic thinking. Emily's reluctance to delegate came from a place of perfectionism—she believed no one else could meet her high standards.

After a particularly overwhelming week, Emily decided to change her approach. She started small, delegating routine tasks like compiling weekly reports and scheduling social media posts. She provided clear instructions and timelines but resisted the urge to micromanage. Over time, Emily's team not only met her expectations but exceeded them. They felt trusted and valued, which boosted their engagement and productivity. Emily, on the other hand, finally had the mental space to focus on long-term projects and innovative ideas. The quality of work improved across the board, demonstrating that delegation isn't just about offloading work—it's about unlocking collective potential.

Key Benefits of Delegation

1. **Increased Efficiency**: Delegating routine or lower-priority tasks frees up your time for strategic, high-impact responsibilities only you can handle. This creates a ripple effect of efficiency across your team.

2. **Empowered Team Members**: Delegation helps others develop new skills, build confidence, and take ownership of their contributions. It fosters a sense of responsibility and pride, leading to stronger collaboration.

3. **Improved Work-Life Balance**: Sharing the workload reduces stress and creates more opportunities for relaxation and self-care, preventing burnout and increasing overall well-being.

4. **Enhanced Team Dynamics**: A culture of shared responsibility strengthens trust, improves communication, and aligns team members toward common goals.

Overcoming Barriers to Delegation

While the benefits of delegation are clear, many struggle with letting go. Here are common barriers and strategies to address them:

1. **Fear of Losing Control**

    o   *Challenge*: "What if the work doesn't meet my standards?"

    o   *Solution*: Start with small, low-risk tasks to build confidence in others. Provide clear guidelines and trust the process.

2. **Doubt in Others' Abilities**

    o   *Challenge*: "No one else can do this as well as I can."

    o   *Solution*: Match tasks to team members' strengths. Use delegation as an opportunity to mentor and develop their skills.

3. **Guilt About Asking for Help**

    o   *Challenge*: "I don't want to burden anyone else."

    o   *Solution*: Recognize that delegation is an opportunity for growth, not a burden. Frame tasks as opportunities for team members to contribute and shine.

Interactive Exercise: Delegation Planner

This activity will help you identify tasks you can delegate and develop a plan for implementation.

1. **Step 1: List Tasks**: Write down 5 tasks you currently handle.

    o   Which of these could be done by someone else?

    o   Which tasks align with others' strengths or goals?

2. **Step 2: Identify Delegates:** For each task, identify a person who could handle it. Consider their skills, workload, and professional development needs.

3. **Step 3: Create Clear Instructions**: For each task, outline:

    o   What needs to be done.

- o Deadlines and priorities.

- o Any resources or support they'll need.

4. **Step 4: Reflect and Plan**

- o What's holding you back from delegating these tasks?

- o How can you overcome these barriers?

- o Set a goal to delegate at least one task this week.

Case Study: The Bakery Turnaround

Javier, a bakery owner, prided himself on overseeing every detail, from sourcing ingredients to decorating cakes. But his 14-hour days were taking a toll. A mentor encouraged him to delegate. Javier started by training a team member to manage inventory and another to oversee customer service. Over time, he empowered his staff to make creative decisions, such as designing new menu items. The bakery thrived, customers loved the fresh ideas, and Javier finally had time to focus on growing the business.

Additional Tips for Effective Delegation

- • **Start Small:** Begin by delegating one or two manageable tasks to build confidence in the process.

- • **Communicate Expectations:** Be specific about goals and deliverables to avoid misunderstandings.

- • **Provide Feedback:** Regularly check in and offer constructive feedback to support learning and improvement.

- • **Celebrate Success:** Acknowledge and celebrate accomplishments to reinforce trust and collaboration.

By embracing delegation, you not only lighten your load but also empower those around you to excel. It's a win-win strategy that fosters collaboration, builds trust, and paves the way for shared success.

6.2 Overcoming Barriers to Delegation

For many, delegation feels like handing over the steering wheel on a winding road—it's uncomfortable and filled with "what ifs." What if the person can't handle it? What if the quality isn't up to par? These fears can create a mental block, keeping you tethered to tasks that could be handled by others. Yet, addressing these barriers head-on can unlock untapped potential in both yourself and your team. Delegation isn't about relinquishing control; it's about creating partnerships, fostering trust, and building a stronger foundation for success. By identifying and overcoming the common obstacles to delegation, you can transform it from a source of stress into a strategy for growth.

Fear of Losing Control

One of the most common barriers to delegation is the belief that only you can execute a task to the highest standard. While this mindset stems from a desire for excellence, it can lead to burnout and inefficiency. The key to overcoming this fear is learning to trust your team and embracing imperfection as part of the growth process.

Case Study: Raj's Perfectionist Trap

Raj, a small business owner, was known for his meticulous approach to every aspect of his company, from product design to customer service. While his dedication was admirable, it also became a bottleneck. Tasks piled up, deadlines were missed, and his employees felt undervalued and underutilized.

Encouraged by a mentor, Raj decided to start delegating smaller, less critical tasks. He trained his team on specific processes, outlined clear expectations, and scheduled weekly check-ins. To his surprise, not only did his team perform well, but they also brought fresh ideas to the table. Delegating allowed Raj to focus on strategic planning, and the overall productivity of his business improved dramatically.

Strategies to Build Trust and Release Control

1. **Start Small**

   o Begin by delegating routine or low-stakes tasks. For example, instead of overseeing daily scheduling, assign it to a trusted team member.

   o Success in smaller tasks will gradually build your confidence in your team's abilities.

2. **Communicate Clearly**

   o Ambiguity leads to errors and frustration. Provide specific instructions, define clear goals, and outline expected outcomes.

   o Example: Instead of saying, "Create a report," specify, "Compile a 2-page summary of this month's sales figures by next Friday."

3. **Check-In Without Micromanaging**

   o Regular updates help ensure progress without undermining your team's autonomy. Ask open-ended questions like, "How is the task progressing?" rather than micromanaging every step.

4. **Acknowledge Success and Provide Feedback**

   o Celebrate completed tasks and provide constructive feedback to support improvement. Recognition boosts morale and reinforces a culture of trust.

Doubt in Others' Abilities

Another barrier is the belief that no one else is capable of performing a task as well as you. While it's natural to take pride in your work, this mindset stifles growth and overlooks the potential of those around you.

Case Study: Grace's Team Transformation

Grace, a nonprofit director, felt overwhelmed by grant-writing responsibilities. She believed no one on her team had the expertise to handle such a nuanced task. At the advice of a leadership coach, Grace provided a team member with templates and guidelines to draft smaller grant applications. Over time, the team member not only mastered the process but also developed innovative strategies that Grace had never considered. This allowed Grace to focus on networking and securing larger grants, which ultimately benefited the organization.

Strategies to Alleviate Doubt:

- **Focus on Development:** Treat delegation as an opportunity for team members to learn and grow. Offer guidance and training where needed.

- **Encourage Initiative:** Allow team members to bring their creativity and problem-solving skills to the task.

- **Reframe Mistakes:** View errors as learning experiences for everyone involved, including yourself.

Interactive Activity: Trust-Building Worksheet

This exercise will help you identify and address your delegation hesitations.

1. **Identify the Task**: Write down one task you've been reluctant to delegate. For example:

   o Task: "Creating the weekly sales report."

2. **Analyze Your Hesitation**: Reflect on why you're hesitant to delegate it.

   o "I worry they won't format it correctly."

   o "I feel it's quicker if I do it myself."

3. **Develop a Delegation Plan**

   o   Choose someone on your team who could take on the task.

   o   Write down clear instructions and expectations for completing it.

   o   Plan a check-in schedule. For example, "Review progress every Wednesday."

4. **Reflect on the Outcome**: After the task is completed, evaluate the results:

   o   Did they meet expectations?

   o   What worked well, and what could be improved?

   o   How did delegating free up your time and energy?

Guilt About Asking for Help

Many people avoid delegation out of fear that they're overburdening others or appearing incapable. However, delegation is not a sign of weakness—it's an opportunity for collaboration and shared success.

Case Study: Daniel's Team Empowerment

Daniel, a high school principal, hesitated to delegate tasks to his already-busy administrative team. But during a leadership workshop, he realized that delegating wasn't just about offloading work; it was about fostering trust and encouraging growth. By assigning projects like organizing school events and managing budgets to his team, Daniel not only lightened his workload but also gave his staff valuable opportunities to develop leadership skills.

Strategies to Reduce Guilt:

- **Reframe Delegation as Empowerment:** Recognize that delegation helps others build skills and confidence.

- **Consider Capacity:** Discuss workload with your team to ensure tasks are distributed fairly.

- **Acknowledge Collaboration:** Emphasize the shared nature of success when goals are achieved.

Interactive Activity: Delegation Confidence Tracker

Use this tracker to measure your delegation progress and build confidence over time.

1. **Start Small:**
   - Week 1: Delegate a simple task.
   - Week 2: Delegate a moderately challenging task.

2. **Track Your Experience:**
   - How did it feel to delegate?
   - What feedback did you receive from the person taking on the task?

3. **Celebrate Wins:**
   - Note the time you saved and how it contributed to your focus on other priorities.
   - Reflect on the growth or new skills demonstrated by your team.

By addressing fears and hesitations head-on, you can transform delegation from a source of anxiety into a tool for empowerment. Letting go of control and trusting others not only lightens your load but also strengthens relationships and fosters a culture of collaboration.

6.3 Building Trust in Relationships

Trust forms the cornerstone of not only effective delegation but also any meaningful relationship—be it personal or professional. It's the invisible thread that holds teams, friendships, and partnerships together, allowing individuals to work in harmony toward shared goals. Building trust takes time and intentional effort, but its rewards are immeasurable: better collaboration, deeper connections, and a more fulfilling sense of mutual respect.

The Layers of Trust

Trust is built incrementally, like layering bricks to construct a solid wall. It begins with consistent actions—following through on commitments and showing reliability. Open communication strengthens these layers, providing a foundation where individuals feel heard and valued. Finally, trust is fortified by moments of vulnerability, where people show authenticity, admit mistakes, and share genuine appreciation.

Case Study: Susan and Her Remote Team

Susan managed a remote team spread across multiple countries and time zones. At first, she struggled to trust that her team members were truly engaged with their work. Productivity felt inconsistent, and she worried about micromanaging. Susan decided to implement weekly video calls where the team could discuss challenges, share goals, and celebrate small wins together. She also began openly recognizing individual contributions through emails and in meetings.

The result? Her team flourished. Members took initiative, collaborated more effectively, and demonstrated a deeper commitment to shared objectives. Susan learned that fostering trust wasn't about constant oversight but creating an environment where her team felt empowered.

Trust-Building Strategies

Consistency Matters

Reliability is the bedrock of trust. Consistently following through on commitments, whether big or small, signals to others that they can depend on you. For example, if you promise a team member you'll review their work by Friday, ensure you do so. This predictability fosters a sense of stability in relationships.

Open Communication

Trust thrives on transparency. Sharing clear expectations, goals, and feedback minimizes misunderstandings and fosters a collaborative environment. Open communication is a two-way street—listening is just as important as sharing. Encouraging honest dialogue, especially about challenges or concerns, strengthens connections and builds mutual respect.

Example: If you're leading a team project, outline the roles and responsibilities for each member at the outset. Then invite input: "Does this align with your strengths? Is there anything you need from me to succeed?"

Recognition and Appreciation

Acknowledging the contributions of others fosters goodwill and reinforces trust. Recognition can be as simple as a "thank you" email or a public acknowledgment during a meeting. These moments show that you value others' efforts, which strengthens their confidence in the relationship.

Example: A manager might say, "Your innovative ideas during last week's brainstorming session significantly shaped the project. Thank you for your contribution!"

Overcoming Trust Barriers

While building trust is essential, rebuilding it after it's broken can be even more critical. Acknowledge missteps openly and commit to corrective actions. For example, if a colleague feels let down by a missed deadline, own up to the mistake and discuss steps to avoid recurrence.

Rebuilding Trust

- **Apologize:** Acknowledge the issue without making excuses.

- **Commit to Change:** Share specific actions you'll take to restore trust.

- **Be Patient:** Understand that rebuilding trust takes time and consistent effort.

Interactive Activities

Trust Reflection Journal

1. **Identify a Relationship:** Think of a personal or professional relationship where trust feels weak or needs improvement.

2. **Assess the Cause:** Reflect on why trust may be lacking. Is it due to past mistakes, misunderstandings, or inconsistent behavior?

3. **Action Plan:** Write down one specific action you can take to rebuild or strengthen trust. For example:

   o Apologizing for a past misstep.

   o Scheduling regular check-ins to show commitment.

   o Being more transparent in your communication.

4. **Track Progress:** Over the next two weeks, observe and journal any changes in the relationship. Reflect on how your actions influence trust and connection.

Trust-Building Challenge

Encourage collaboration in a group setting by assigning tasks that require teamwork and interdependence.

1. Divide participants into small groups.

2. Give each group a task where success hinges on relying on each other's strengths. For example, solving a problem or completing a creative project.

3. Afterward, discuss how trust influenced the outcome:

   o How did you rely on your teammates?

   o Were there moments where trust felt tested?

   o How did the experience shape your perception of the group?

Building trust is a process of steady effort and genuine care. It requires showing up consistently, communicating openly, and celebrating the contributions of others. When trust flourishes, so do relationships, making delegation and collaboration more seamless and rewarding. As you strengthen trust in your personal and professional life, you'll create a foundation for deeper connections and greater success.

6.4 Letting Go: Embracing Imperfection in Others

Imagine walking through a garden filled with diverse blooms—some vibrant and sprawling, others delicate and understated. Each flower adds its unique beauty to the landscape, thriving in its own time and way. Similarly, when we embrace the imperfections of those around us, we create an environment where growth, creativity, and harmony can flourish.

Letting go of the need for others to meet rigid standards isn't about lowering expectations; it's about recognizing that perfection isn't a prerequisite for value. Accepting others as they are fosters trust, strengthens relationships, and unlocks the potential for collaboration and innovation.

Case Study: Marco's Micromanagement Shift

Marco, a marketing team leader, struggled with relinquishing control. He believed his way of working was the most efficient and insisted his team adhere to his methods. This approach stifled creativity, leaving team members frustrated and disengaged. After attending a leadership workshop, Marco had an epiphany: his need for control was holding his team back.

He began encouraging team members to present their ideas and explore new approaches, even if it meant making mistakes. Over time, Marco's team felt empowered to take risks and innovate. The result? They delivered some of their most successful campaigns, each marked by the unique contributions of the team.

Key Takeaway: Letting go of rigid control doesn't mean compromising standards. It means trusting others to bring their strengths to the table.

Empathy in Action

Empathy is the cornerstone of embracing imperfection. By putting yourself in someone else's shoes, you develop a deeper understanding of their perspective, challenges, and strengths. This connection fosters mutual respect and collaboration.

Practical Steps to Cultivate Empathy:

1. **Active Listening:** Pay full attention when someone is speaking. Resist the urge to interrupt or formulate your response while they talk.

2. **Ask Open-Ended Questions:** Encourage dialogue by asking questions that invite detailed responses. For example, "Can you tell me more about how you approached that challenge?"

3. **Acknowledge Their Feelings:** Use phrases like, "That sounds really challenging," or, "I can see how much effort you put into this."

Interactive Activity: Empathy Challenge

1. **Choose a Day:** Spend one day actively practicing empathy with everyone you interact with—whether at work, home, or in social settings.

2. **Observe and Record:** After each interaction, jot down insights about the person's perspective or emotions that you might not have noticed before.

3. **Reflect:** How did this practice change the dynamic of your interactions? What new understanding did you gain about the people around you?

This challenge helps build the habit of empathy, creating stronger connections and a more inclusive environment.

Managing Expectations

Balancing flexibility with clear guidelines allows others to grow without the fear of being judged harshly. Establishing realistic expectations fosters trust and sets a foundation for success.

Case Study: Sofia's Creative Team

Sofia managed a group of instructional designers who often felt stifled by her strict deadlines and exacting standards. Realizing her approach was hindering the team's creativity, Sofia started setting broader goals with reasonable timelines. She encouraged her team to innovate on course materials and approaches, providing constructive feedback along the way. She encouraged her team to experiment with their designs, providing constructive feedback along the way. The result? The team's creativity soared, producing innovative and high-quality work that exceeded expectations.

Strategies for Managing Expectations:

1. **Communicate Clearly:** Outline goals and objectives while leaving room for individual interpretation.

2. **Encourage Flexibility:** Accept that processes may vary and allow for creative problem-solving.

3. **Celebrate Effort and Progress:** Recognize milestones along the way, not just the final outcome.

Letting go of the need for perfection in others allows creativity, trust, and collaboration to flourish. By practicing empathy, managing expectations, and encouraging a growth mindset, you create an environment where everyone—including yourself—can thrive. The freedom to embrace imperfection not only strengthens relationships but also opens the door to innovation and mutual success.

The Psychological Benefits of Letting Go

Letting go of control not only improves efficiency and collaboration but also enhances your mental and emotional well-being. Research shows that relinquishing the need for control reduces stress and fosters a sense of empowerment in others. It creates opportunities for creativity and innovation, as team members feel free to experiment and take risks.

Case Study: Jacob's Innovative Breakthrough

Jacob, a tech startup founder, was known for micromanaging every detail of product development. When his workload became unmanageable, he reluctantly handed over some responsibilities to his lead developer. The result? The developer introduced a feature that became the company's most popular product. By stepping back, Jacob allowed his team to shine and discovered the power of collaboration.

Interactive Activities to Let Go of Control

1. The Delegation Experiment

- Choose one task you typically micromanage.

- Delegate it to a team member, providing only the necessary instructions.

- Avoid intervening unless absolutely necessary.

- Reflect on the outcome: Did the world fall apart? What did you learn about your team's capabilities?

2. Visualize Your Ideal Role

- Close your eyes and imagine yourself as a leader or collaborator who trusts others completely.

- What tasks are you focusing on?

- How does it feel to let go of smaller responsibilities?

- Write down one step you can take to move closer to this ideal.

3. Mindfulness Practice for Letting Go

- Spend five minutes each day practicing mindfulness.

- Focus on your breath and observe any thoughts about control without judgment.

- Over time, this practice will help you recognize and release the need for control in the moment.

Final Reflection

Delegation and trust are not about relinquishing responsibility but about sharing it wisely. Letting go of the need to control everything allows others to contribute, fosters innovation, and builds stronger relationships. It also liberates you from unnecessary stress, enabling you to focus on what truly matters.

Action Step: Reflect on one area in your life where you feel overly controlling. What is one small action you can take this week to relinquish control and empower someone else? Write it down and commit to following through.

Looking Ahead

As you practice letting go and embracing imperfection, you'll find greater freedom, balance, and fulfillment. In the next chapter, we will explore how procrastination feeds into perfectionism and how to break the cycle to reclaim your time and focus.

Procrastination and Perfectionism

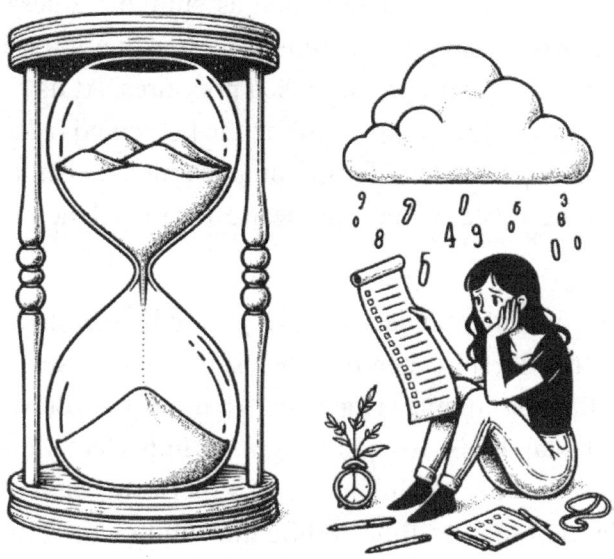

Think about standing in front of a blank canvas, brush in hand, yet hesitating to make the first stroke. The fear of not creating a masterpiece prevents you from starting at all. This hesitation, familiar to many perfectionists, highlights how the pursuit of perfection often leads to procrastination. The fear of falling short of lofty standards can paralyze you, creating a cycle of avoidance and delay. It's not about laziness but the overwhelming weight of expectations—both self-imposed and external.

This chapter explores the intricate connection between perfectionism and procrastination, offering practical strategies to disrupt this cycle. By understanding the psychological underpinnings and embracing actionable steps, you can transform hesitation into progress, allowing your creativity and productivity to flourish.

7.1 Understanding the Connection Between Procrastination and Perfectionism

Procrastination is often misunderstood as simple laziness or lack of motivation. However, for perfectionists, procrastination is deeply tied to psychological fears and self-imposed pressures. At its core, it's not about avoiding work but about avoiding the perceived risks associated with failure or imperfection. This avoidance mechanism can become a self-sabotaging cycle, where the desire for excellence stalls action altogether.

For instance, consider Dylan, a college student with a knack for creative writing. Despite her passion, she finds herself putting off essays until the last minute. Her fear? That her first draft won't live up to her high standards. Instead of writing imperfectly and revising, Dylan delays starting, believing she'll perform better under the pressure of a looming deadline. While this might work temporarily, it reinforces a pattern that leaves her feeling stressed and dissatisfied.

Exploring Psychological Roots

Let's delve deeper into some psychological underpinnings that contribute to procrastination:

- **Temporal Discounting:** This psychological concept highlights how people tend to value immediate comfort more than distant rewards. For perfectionists, the discomfort of starting a task (and potentially making mistakes) feels more urgent than the satisfaction of finishing it. This results in prioritizing short-term relief over long-term achievement.

- **Task Aversion:** Tasks that seem complex, ambiguous, or likely to highlight perceived inadequacies are often avoided. For example, writing a report or delivering a presentation may

141

feel overwhelming because of the high standards set internally.

- **Fear of Judgment:** Perfectionists often internalize the fear of how others might perceive their work. This leads to delaying tasks as a way of postponing potential criticism.

Procrastination Behaviors in Action

The behaviors of procrastination vary but share common threads of avoidance. Here's how they typically manifest:

- **Excessive Planning:** Planning is a necessary part of achieving goals, but for perfectionists, it can turn into a form of avoidance. For instance, instead of starting an assignment, one might spend hours creating color-coded schedules and detailed outlines without making tangible progress.

- **Waiting for Perfect Conditions:** Perfectionists often convince themselves that they'll start once "the time is right." Whether it means the need for absolute silence, a completely clean workspace, or all resources perfectly aligned, this waiting game becomes a stalling tactic.

- **Analysis Paralysis:** Overanalyzing options or potential outcomes can lead to complete inaction. This is particularly common when faced with decisions that have no objectively perfect answer, such as choosing between two viable strategies.

Emotional Consequences of Procrastination

The emotional toll of procrastination is significant and often exacerbates the perfectionist tendencies that caused the delay in the first place.

- **Guilt and Anxiety:** As deadlines approach, the knowledge of tasks left undone builds stress and regret. This is often compounded by self-recrimination, as perfectionists blame themselves for the delay.

- **Negative Self-Perception:** Procrastination can create a vicious cycle of self-doubt. The more a person delays, the more they see themselves as someone who cannot meet their own standards, which fuels further procrastination.

Case Study: Navigating Procrastination as a New Manager

Jennifer, a newly promoted manager, found herself struggling with procrastination when drafting performance reviews for her team. She feared that her feedback wouldn't be insightful enough, which led her to delay the task repeatedly. As the deadline loomed, she hastily completed the reviews, leaving her feeling rushed and dissatisfied.

By identifying her triggers—fear of not meeting her own high expectations and discomfort with giving feedback—Jennifer began to implement small changes. She broke the task into smaller steps, writing one review at a time and seeking input from a mentor. Over time, she learned to focus on the progress she was making rather than the unattainable ideal of "perfect" reviews.

Interactive Activity: Procrastination Triggers Journal

Take some time to reflect on your own procrastination habits. Answer the following prompts in a dedicated journal:

1. **Task Patterns:** What types of tasks do you procrastinate on most frequently? (e.g., creative projects, administrative tasks, personal goals)

2. **Underlying Beliefs:** What fears or beliefs might be contributing to your procrastination? Examples could include fear of failure, fear of judgment, or perfectionist tendencies.

3. **Emotional Impact:** How does procrastination affect your emotions and overall mindset? (e.g., Does it make you feel guilty, anxious, or overwhelmed?)

4. **Past Patterns:** Reflect on a time when procrastination impacted an important goal. What was the outcome, and what might you have done differently?

This journaling exercise provides clarity on your procrastination patterns, helping you identify specific areas for improvement.

Exercises and Strategies to Manage Procrastination

- **"Just 5 Minutes" Strategy:** Commit to working on a task for just five minutes. Often, starting is the hardest part, and this approach helps you overcome the initial resistance.

- **Procrastination-Free Zones:** Designate specific times and places as "procrastination-free zones" where you work without distractions. This could mean turning off your phone, clearing your workspace, or setting a timer.

- **Create an Imperfect Start Challenge:** Choose a task you've been avoiding and challenge yourself to start imperfectly. For example, write the messiest first draft possible or sketch a quick outline for a project. The goal is to prioritize progress over perfection.

- **Visualization Exercise:** Close your eyes and visualize completing the task. Imagine how it feels to finish and the relief or pride that comes with it. Write down the steps needed to reach that outcome.

Expanding Awareness

Understanding the connection between procrastination and perfectionism is the first step in breaking free from their grip. By recognizing how psychological tendencies, like task aversion and temporal discounting, play a role, you gain insight into your own behaviors. Coupling this awareness with practical tools like journaling, visualization, and structured approaches creates a path to action. As you delve deeper into these strategies, you'll discover that overcoming procrastination is less about achieving perfection and more about embracing the value of starting and finishing with purpose.

7.2 Breaking the Procrastination Cycle

Breaking the procrastination cycle requires intentional strategies that address both the emotional and practical barriers keeping tasks unfinished. Procrastination isn't just a lack of time management or motivation—it often stems from deeper fears, self-doubt, or perfectionist tendencies that can feel overwhelming. To overcome this pattern, it's essential to recognize that procrastination is a behavior that can be reshaped, not an inherent flaw.

By identifying the root causes of procrastination and implementing targeted strategies, you can begin to break free from the grip of avoidance. Effective techniques, such as time management tools, mental reframing, and structured accountability, provide a roadmap for taking action. Each step, no matter how small, contributes to momentum and builds confidence in your ability to tackle tasks head-on.

Furthermore, transforming procrastination into productive action involves cultivating a mindset that values progress over perfection. This shift not only reduces the fear of starting but also fosters a sense of accomplishment with each completed step. With the right strategies and a willingness to reframe negative thought patterns, breaking free from the cycle of procrastination becomes an achievable and empowering process. This section delves into actionable tools and insights that help dismantle the barriers to productivity, paving the way for meaningful progress.

Techniques to Interrupt the Cycle

Implementing practical strategies can help disrupt the habitual patterns of procrastination. These tools provide structure, reduce overwhelm, and create momentum.

- **Timeboxing:** This method involves allocating specific time blocks for tasks. For instance, if you're hesitant to start writing a report, set a timer for 30 minutes and focus solely on writing during that time. Knowing the task has a defined endpoint reduces the anxiety of endless effort and helps you initiate action.

- **The Pomodoro Technique:** Break your work into 25-minute intervals followed by a 5-minute break. This technique creates a sense of urgency and rewards focus with frequent breaks, making even large tasks feel manageable. After four cycles, take a longer break of 15-30 minutes to recharge. For perfectionists, the predefined intervals can help counteract the tendency to overwork on minor details.

- **Prioritization with Deadlines:** Tools like the Eisenhower Matrix allow you to categorize tasks based on urgency and importance:

  - **Urgent and Important:** Handle these tasks first.

  - **Important but Not Urgent:** Schedule these for later.

  - **Urgent but Not Important:** Delegate these tasks.

  - **Neither Urgent Nor Important:** Consider eliminating these tasks.

This approach helps perfectionists focus on what truly matters rather than getting bogged down in unimportant details.

Expanded Techniques for Progress

- **Micro-Steps Approach:** Break tasks into the smallest possible steps. For example, instead of writing "finish presentation" on your to-do list, start with "create title slide." Small wins build momentum and reduce the intimidation of large tasks.

- **Pre-Task Rituals:** Create a ritual to signal the start of focused work. This might include a short mindfulness exercise, organizing your workspace, or setting up a timer. These cues prepare your mind for productivity.

- **Mind Mapping:** Visualize your task using a mind map. Write the main goal in the center and branch out with smaller steps or ideas. This method reduces overwhelm by creating a clear, visual roadmap.

Cognitive-Behavioral Strategies

Addressing the thought patterns underlying procrastination is key to breaking the cycle.

- **Identify and Challenge Negative Thoughts:** Many perfectionists struggle with internal dialogue that predicts failure or inadequacy. When you catch yourself thinking, "I'll never finish this," challenge the thought by asking, "What evidence supports this?" Replace it with, "Every small step I take moves me closer to my goal."

- **Reframe Perfection:** Replace the fear of imperfection with a focus on progress. Remind yourself that "done is better than perfect" and that you can always refine your work later if needed.

- **Visualizing Outcomes:** Imagine the benefits of completing your task. Visualize yourself meeting the deadline, feeling accomplished, and freeing up time for other priorities. This positive reinforcement can motivate you to take the first step.

Interactive Exercises

1. **Timeboxing Challenge**

   o Choose a task you've been procrastinating on.

   o Set a timer for 20-30 minutes and commit to working on it during that time.

o After the timer ends, assess your progress and take a short break. Repeat as needed.

o Reflect: Did the time constraint help you focus? Write down what worked and any challenges you faced.

2. **Reframing Thoughts Worksheet**

o Write down three negative thoughts you often have about starting a task (e.g., "I'll never get it right").

o Challenge each thought by writing evidence that disproves it.

o Replace the negative thought with a positive or neutral statement (e.g., "I can make progress, even if it's small").

3. **Accountability Planner**

o List three tasks you've been putting off.

o Identify an accountability partner for each task and schedule a check-in date.

o Track your progress and discuss outcomes during the check-ins.

4. **Procrastination Diary**

o For one week, log moments when you procrastinate. Include:

  ▪ The task you avoided.

  ▪ How you felt emotionally.

  ▪ What you did instead.

o Review the diary at the end of the week to identify patterns and triggers. Use these insights to create a plan for tackling similar situations.

Breaking the procrastination cycle requires a mix of practical techniques, cognitive shifts, and external support. By implementing strategies like timeboxing, reframing negative thoughts, and leveraging accountability, you can take control of your productivity and reduce the stress associated with procrastination. Remember, progress is more important than perfection, and every small step forward is a step toward reclaiming your time and energy.

7.3 Actionable Steps to Start and Finish Tasks

Facing a daunting task can feel like standing at the base of a mountain, unsure where to begin or how to reach the top. The key to overcoming this initial inertia is developing actionable strategies that transform overwhelming projects into manageable, achievable steps. Starting and finishing tasks isn't just about discipline; it's about creating an environment and mindset that support progress. By breaking tasks into smaller pieces, maintaining momentum through checkpoints and rewards, and building consistent work habits, you can turn procrastination into productivity. This section explores practical tools and techniques to help you start tasks with confidence and follow through to completion.

Breaking Tasks Into Manageable Pieces

Large tasks can seem paralyzing when viewed as a whole. By dividing them into smaller, more specific steps, you can reduce the sense of overwhelm and create a clear path forward. This method provides a roadmap, helping you focus on one step at a time rather than the entire journey.

Example:

Suppose you're tasked with writing a detailed report. Breaking it into steps might look like this:

- **Research:** Gather and organize relevant sources.

- **Draft Key Sections:** Focus on one section at a time, such as the introduction, body, or conclusion.

- **Editing:** Review for clarity, grammar, and coherence.

By focusing on one phase at a time, the project becomes more approachable, and each completed step builds momentum for the next.

Building Consistent Work Habit:

Habits create structure and reduce the mental effort required to begin tasks. Developing consistent routines helps you establish a rhythm that supports productivity.

- **Routine Matters:** Dedicate specific times for focused work. For instance, reserve mornings for creative tasks when your mind is fresh, and afternoons for administrative or routine activities.

- **Batch Similar Tasks:** Group related activities, such as responding to emails or organizing files, to maintain a flow state and minimize transitions between tasks.

Example:

Mark, a marketing professional, started batching his daily tasks—responding to emails from 9:00 to 9:30 a.m. and reserving the next two hours for strategic planning. This streamlined approach improved his efficiency and reduced decision fatigue.

Interactive Activity: Task Visualization

Visualization is a powerful tool for overcoming procrastination and building confidence.

Instructions:

1. Choose a task you've been avoiding.

2. Close your eyes and visualize completing it successfully.

o Picture each step you'll take.

o Imagine the sense of accomplishment when the task is finished.

o Focus on the benefits this completion will bring.

3. Write down this mental roadmap, breaking it into actionable steps.

4. Use this guide as a starting point to take your first small step.

Example:

If the task is organizing your workspace, visualize the process step by step: clearing the clutter, sorting items into categories, and arranging essentials for easy access. Imagine how satisfying it will feel to have a clean, functional area to work in. Write down these steps and commit to starting the process immediately.

By integrating these actionable steps into your daily routine, you can create a structure that supports both starting and finishing tasks. Breaking tasks into manageable pieces, maintaining momentum with rewards, and building productive habits will empower you to tackle challenges with confidence. With practice, these strategies will help you approach tasks with clarity and purpose, turning daunting projects into opportunities for achievement.

7.4 Maintaining Focus Amidst Distractions

In a world brimming with distractions, maintaining focus has become a skill as essential as the tasks themselves. From the constant buzz of digital notifications to the chaos of a cluttered workspace, distractions can derail even the most disciplined among us. For perfectionists, who often strive for an ideal work environment or outcome, distractions can feel particularly overwhelming. Learning to manage these interruptions and cultivate an environment conducive to focus is key to overcoming procrastination and achieving meaningful progress.

Identifying Common Distractions

To maintain focus, you must first identify the specific distractions that challenge your productivity. Understanding these interruptions helps you create targeted strategies to address them.

- **Digital Distractions:** Social media notifications, email alerts, and text messages pull your attention away from tasks. The lure of endless scrolling or checking your inbox can fragment focus and disrupt workflow.

- **Environmental Distractions:** A cluttered desk, background noise, or interruptions from others can make it hard to concentrate. Visual or auditory chaos often mirrors internal disorganization, amplifying the challenge of staying on track.

- **Internal Distractions:** Mental clutter, like overthinking or daydreaming, can also hinder focus. Thoughts about other tasks, personal concerns, or perfectionist tendencies to plan excessively may divert your attention.

Case Study:

Lisa, an engineer, found herself constantly interrupted by notifications during her workday. Despite having set deadlines, she struggled to complete projects on time. After tracking her distractions, she realized that checking emails and social media consumed nearly two hours daily. By identifying this pattern, Lisa took the first step toward regaining her focus.

Strategies to Stay Focused

Once you've pinpointed your distractions, implementing effective strategies can help you regain control over your attention and productivity.

- **Create a Distraction-Free Zone:** Dedicate a specific area for focused work. Keep this space organized, clutter-free, and stocked with essentials to reduce the temptation to leave for non-work-related reasons. Turn off non-essential notifications, set your phone to "Do Not Disturb," and use tools like website blockers to prevent digital interruptions.

- **Mindfulness Breaks:** Integrate short mindfulness sessions throughout your day to reset and refocus. Simple exercises, such as taking five deep breaths or practicing a two-minute meditation, can help clear mental clutter and bring your attention back to the task.

- **Time Management Tools:** Use productivity apps like Focus@Will or techniques like the Pomodoro Technique to create structured work periods interspersed with short breaks. These methods help maintain momentum while preventing burnout.

Managing External Interruptions

External interruptions can often feel out of your control, but proactive measures can minimize their impact.

- **Set Boundaries:** Clearly communicate your need for uninterrupted work time to colleagues, family, or housemates. Establish specific work hours and use visual cues, such as a closed door or a "Do Not Disturb" sign, to signal when you need focus.

- **Prepare for Interruptions:** Plan responses for potential distractions. For example, if a colleague frequently stops by your desk, prepare a polite script to redirect them, such as, "I'd love to discuss this later, but I need to finish something right now."

- **Delegate or Delay Non-Urgent Requests:** Learn to prioritize interruptions. If a request can wait, schedule it for a more convenient time instead of allowing it to derail your current task.

Case Study:

Callum, a remote worker, struggled with interruptions from his young children during work hours. By setting clear boundaries and scheduling focused work periods during their nap times, he created a more productive work environment while still being present for his family.

Interactive Element: Personal Focus Plan

Developing a personalized focus plan helps you integrate focus-enhancing strategies into your daily routine.

Instructions:

1. **Create a Daily Checklist:**
   o   Set up your workspace each morning.
   o   Identify potential distractions and strategies to address them.
   o   Plan mindfulness breaks.
   o   Implement digital detox practices (e.g., turning off notifications, using a focus app).

2. **Track Your Progress**: At the end of each day, review your checklist to assess how well you maintained focus and where improvements can be made.

3. **Refine Your Plan**: Adjust your checklist based on what worked and what didn't. For instance, if you find that digital detox practices are highly effective, allocate more time to these strategies.

Example Checklist:

- Declutter workspace.
- Turn off phone notifications.
- Schedule three mindfulness breaks.
- Use the Pomodoro Technique for focused work.

Closing Reflections: From Procrastination to Progress

Maintaining focus amidst distractions is an ongoing practice that requires self-awareness and intentionality. By addressing common interruptions, creating distraction-free environments, and setting clear boundaries, you pave the way for consistent progress. Remember that focus is a muscle—one that strengthens with practice and perseverance.

Mindfulness and Stress Reduction

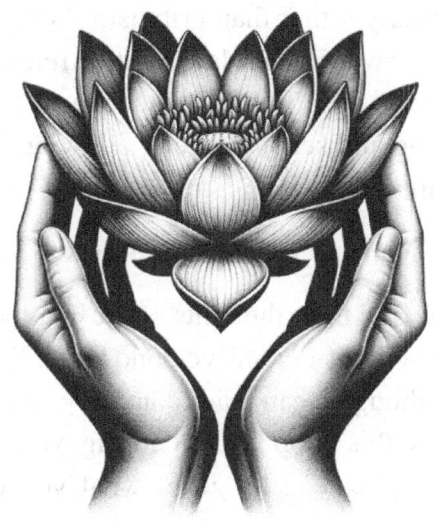

Try to see yourself standing in the center of a whirlwind. Tasks fly around you, each shouting for attention, yet your ability to focus feels stretched thin, and your thoughts dart from one worry to the next. For many, this is the everyday reality of perfectionism—a relentless loop of overthinking and self-criticism. In these moments, mindfulness offers a powerful reprieve: a quiet space where you can step back, observe, and find calm. By practicing mindfulness, you shift from reacting to life's demands to responding with intention. Like clouds drifting through the sky, your thoughts and worries become temporary, not defining truths. Mindfulness replaces perfectionist rigidity with a gentler, more forgiving way of being, helping you rediscover clarity and balance.

8.1 Understanding Mindfulness: A New Way to Approach Perfectionism

Mindfulness is more than a buzzword; it's a transformative way of relating to yourself and the world. At its heart, mindfulness means being fully present in the moment, observing your thoughts and emotions with curiosity rather than criticism. For perfectionists, this practice can be a powerful antidote to the relentless pressure of achieving flawlessness. Mindfulness teaches you to detach from the cycle of overthinking and self-judgment, allowing space for growth, creativity, and balance.

Why Mindfulness Matters for Perfectionists

Perfectionists often find their thoughts stuck in a loop of past regrets or future worries. "What if I could've done better?" or "What if I fail next time?" These thoughts can lead to anxiety, stress, and paralysis. Mindfulness breaks this loop by anchoring your attention in the present moment, helping you let go of what you can't control and focus on what truly matters.

By adopting mindfulness, perfectionists learn to:

- Recognize unhelpful thought patterns.
- Respond to challenges with clarity instead of emotional reactivity.
- Embrace imperfection as part of the human experience.

Expanded Case Study: Amanda's Mindful Shift

Amanda, an event planner, was known for her stunning work but constantly felt drained by her perfectionism. She would obsess over the smallest details, spending hours revising projects that were already excellent. This habit caused her to miss deadlines and feel resentful toward her work.

After attending a mindfulness workshop, Amanda began practicing 10-minute mindfulness sessions each morning. She started by focusing on her breath and observing her thoughts without judgment. Over a few weeks, Amanda noticed a profound change. She approached her designs with curiosity, reminding herself that "done is better than perfect." This mindset helped her meet deadlines, reignite her creative passion, and reduce her work-related anxiety.

Key Benefits of Mindfulness for Perfectionists

1. **Reduced Anxiety**

   o Mindfulness helps you observe your thoughts without attaching emotional weight to them. Instead of spiraling into "what-ifs," you can acknowledge the thought and move on. This practice reduces the emotional intensity of perfectionist thinking, creating a sense of calm.

2. **Increased Self-Acceptance**

   o By observing your inner dialogue without judgment, you begin to see imperfections as natural rather than flaws. This shift fosters a kinder, more compassionate relationship with yourself.

3. **Improved Focus**

   o Staying present allows you to direct your energy toward what truly matters, rather than being bogged down by worries about past mistakes or future outcomes.

Mindfulness offers a powerful way to address the root causes of perfectionism. By observing your thoughts without judgment, focusing on the present, and embracing imperfections, you can transform your relationship with yourself and the world. Remember, mindfulness is not about achieving a perfectly calm state—it's about being present with whatever arises and approaching life with curiosity and compassion. In the next section, we'll explore mindfulness techniques specifically designed to help you manage stress and find moments of peace amidst the chaos.

8.2 Mindfulness Techniques for Stress Relief

Stress and perfectionism often intertwine, feeding off each other to create a cycle of overwhelm. Mindfulness offers a toolkit to break this cycle, helping you calm the storm and approach challenges with clarity and ease. These techniques not only reduce stress but also foster emotional resilience, enabling you to navigate life's demands with greater composure.

Expanded Techniques for Stress Relief

Body Scan Meditation

This foundational mindfulness practice encourages you to tune into your body, noticing sensations without judgment and releasing accumulated tension.

- **How to Practice:**

  1. Lie or sit in a comfortable position in a quiet space.

  2. Close your eyes and take a few deep breaths.

  3. Starting at your toes, slowly focus your attention on each body part, moving upward through your legs, torso, arms, and finally your head.

  4. At each stop, notice sensations such as tightness, tingling, or relaxation.

  5. Imagine exhaling tension with each breath as you progress through the body.

- **Why It Works:** By shifting your focus to the physical body, the practice anchors you in the present moment, reducing mental chatter and stress. It fosters a deeper connection to your physical self, creating a sense of grounding and calm.

- **Case Study: Lydia's Midday Reset** Lydia, a nurse juggling long shifts, often felt overwhelmed by midday. She began practicing a 10-minute body scan during her lunch breaks. This quick reset helped her release physical tension and return to work feeling refreshed and focused.

Guided Imagery

This practice uses visualization to create a mental escape, transporting you to a place of calm and relaxation.

- **How to Practice:**
    1. Close your eyes and imagine a serene location, such as a tranquil forest or a peaceful beach.
    2. Engage all your senses: visualize the sights, hear the sounds, and feel the textures of this place.
    3. Spend 5–10 minutes immersed in this mental space, allowing it to soothe your mind.
- **Why It Works:** Guided imagery provides a mental sanctuary, allowing your brain to rest and reset. It's particularly effective for reducing anxiety and promoting a sense of safety.
- **Interactive Exercise: Your Calm Oasis** On a piece of paper, describe your ideal calming environment in vivid detail. Revisit this imagery during moments of stress for a personalized retreat.

Mindful Breathing

Focusing on the breath is a simple yet powerful way to interrupt stress and return to the present moment.

- **How to Practice:**

    1. Sit comfortably and place one hand on your chest and the other on your belly.

    2. Inhale deeply through your nose, allowing your belly to rise.

    3. Exhale slowly through your mouth, feeling your belly fall.

    4. Repeat for 3–5 minutes, focusing solely on the rhythm of your breath.

- **Why It Works:** Deep breathing activates the parasympathetic nervous system, the body's natural relaxation response. It reduces heart rate, lowers blood pressure, and calms the mind.

- **Case Study: Brett's Pre-Presentation Calm** Brett, a marketing executive, dreaded public speaking. Before his presentations, he practiced mindful breathing for five minutes. This ritual helped him center himself, reducing his nerves and improving his focus.

Movement-Based Mindfulness

Incorporating mindfulness into physical activities such as yoga or walking combines movement with mental presence.

- **How to Practice Mindful Walking:**

    1. Choose a quiet path and walk slowly, focusing on the sensation of your feet touching the ground.

    2. Pay attention to your surroundings—the sound of birds, the feel of the breeze, or the texture of the ground beneath your shoes.

    3. Sync your breathing with your steps to enhance the connection.

- **Why It Works:** Movement-based mindfulness engages both body and mind, offering a holistic way to reduce stress while staying active.

- **Interactive Activity: Movement Journal** After a mindful walk or yoga session, write down three observations you made during the practice. Reflect on how it affected your mood and energy.

STOP Technique

This quick mindfulness tool helps you pause, recalibrate, and respond thoughtfully rather than react impulsively during stressful moments.

- **How to Practice:**
    1. **Stop:** Pause whatever you are doing.
    2. **Take a Breath:** Inhale deeply, focusing on the sensation of the breath entering and leaving your body.
    3. **Observe:** Notice your thoughts, emotions, and body sensations with an open and nonjudgmental mindset.
    4. **Proceed:** Move forward with intention and awareness.

- **Why It Works:** STOP creates a moment of mindfulness amid chaos, breaking the cycle of automatic stress responses.

- **Case Study: Savannah's Conflict Reset** During a heated work discussion, Savannah felt her stress escalating. She practiced the STOP technique, which allowed her to approach the conversation calmly and constructively, leading to a better resolution.

Integrating Techniques into Your Routine

Daily Stress Check-Ins

Incorporate a 2-minute mindfulness break into your day:

- Morning: Begin with 3 deep breaths before starting work.

- Midday: Take a mindful moment during lunch to check in with your body and mind.

- Evening: Reflect on your day with gratitude and deep breathing before bed.

Interactive Workbook Add-On: Stress Tracker

Create a chart to track your stress levels before and after trying a mindfulness practice. Include columns for the date, stress level (on a scale of 1–10), the technique used, and how you felt afterward.

By exploring and incorporating these mindfulness techniques, you can build a personalized toolkit for managing stress effectively. Each method invites you to connect with the present moment, fostering a sense of calm and resilience in the face of life's challenges.

8.3 Staying Present in a Fast-Paced World

In a world of constant notifications, endless to-do lists, and societal pressure to stay "plugged in," staying present can feel like a Herculean task. The digital age offers incredible conveniences, but it also pulls your focus in countless directions, leaving you feeling scattered and disconnected. Mindful practices provide a lifeline, helping you reclaim focus, engage with the moment, and find joy in the here and now.

Understanding the Cost of Distraction

The constant pull of digital distractions doesn't just affect productivity—it impacts mental well-being, relationships, and overall satisfaction. Studies have shown that frequent multitasking increases stress, diminishes memory, and reduces the ability to engage deeply in any one activity. Recognizing this cost is the first step toward reclaiming your presence.

Case Study: Jake's Digital Detox

Jake, a software developer, noticed he spent hours jumping between coding, emails, and social media. He often ended his day feeling exhausted and unaccomplished. After implementing mindful practices like designated screen-free times and single-tasking, Jake's productivity soared. More importantly, he felt calmer and more in control of his day.

Takeaway: Being constantly connected doesn't equal being productive. Disconnecting intentionally allows for more meaningful connections with your tasks and relationships.

The Power of Single-Tasking

Single-tasking involves focusing your full attention on one activity at a time, enhancing both the quality of your work and your enjoyment of the process.

How to Practice Single-Tasking:

1. **Choose One Task:** Identify a priority task and set clear boundaries for your focus.

2. **Eliminate Distractions:** Silence notifications, close unrelated tabs, and set your phone aside.

3. **Use Time Blocks:** Utilize the Pomodoro Technique, dedicating 25 minutes to focused work, followed by a 5-minute break.

4. **Reflect:** After completing the session, evaluate your progress and sense of accomplishment.

Example: Focused Work with the Pomodoro Technique

Working on a report? Close your email, set a timer for 25 minutes, and focus solely on writing. Afterward, take a short break to refresh your mind before diving back in.

Outcome: Improved efficiency, deeper engagement, and reduced mental fatigue.

Practicing Mindful Technology Use

Technology is a double-edged sword: it can either enhance your life or dominate it. Learning to use it mindfully ensures it serves you rather than the other way around.

Strategies for Digital Mindfulness:

1. **Designated Screen-Free Times:** Set specific hours, such as during meals or the first hour after waking, to be tech-free.

2. **Turn Off Non-Essential Notifications:** Reserve your attention for what truly matters.

3. **Digital Detox Days:** Dedicate one day a month to being completely unplugged.

Interactive Exercise: Notification Audit

Spend a day observing how often notifications interrupt your focus. At the end of the day, adjust your settings to minimize unnecessary disruptions.

Mindful Presence in Daily Life

Staying present doesn't require monumental changes. Everyday activities offer opportunities for mindfulness.

Mindful Eating:

- Sit down to a meal without distractions like TV or your phone.

- Pay attention to the textures, tastes, and scents of every bite.

- Chew slowly, savoring the experience.

Outcome: Enhanced enjoyment of food and a healthier relationship with eating.

Deep Listening:

- When engaging in conversations, resist the urge to interrupt or plan your response.

- Focus fully on the speaker's words, tone, and body language.

- Repeat what you've heard to ensure mutual understanding.

Outcome: Improved communication, stronger connections, and a greater sense of empathy.

Mindful Walking:

- Take a short walk outdoors, paying attention to each step.

- Notice the sensation of your feet meeting the ground, the rhythm of your breath, and the sights and sounds around you.

- Use this time as a moving meditation to ground yourself.

Outcome: Reduced stress and a sense of connection to the present moment.

Overcoming Challenges to Staying Present

Challenge: Feeling Overwhelmed by Multitasking

- **Solution:** Start small. Practice single-tasking for just one task each day. Gradually extend this practice as you grow more comfortable.

Challenge: Constant Digital Interruptions

- **Solution:** Create tech boundaries by turning off notifications and setting specific times to check emails and messages.

Challenge: Difficulty Slowing Down

- **Solution:** Integrate micro-mindfulness practices, like taking three deep breaths before transitioning between tasks or meetings.

Interactive Tools for Presence

Presence Tracker Worksheet

- Track moments when you feel present during the day.

- Note the activity, what helped you stay focused, and how it felt.

Mindful Pause Cards

- Create small cards with prompts like "Take a breath," "What do you hear?" or "Focus on one task." Keep these at your desk or in your pocket for quick reminders.

By incorporating these mindful practices into your daily routine, you'll find it easier to stay present even in a fast-paced world. These strategies not only reduce stress but also enrich your experiences, helping you engage more deeply with the people and tasks that matter most. Each small step toward mindfulness creates ripple effects, transforming how you approach both work and life.

8.4 Integrating Mindfulness into Your Daily Routines

Making mindfulness a habit doesn't require major lifestyle changes—it's about weaving small moments of awareness into your day. By building mindfulness into your existing routines, you can experience its benefits without feeling overwhelmed. Each moment of mindfulness is an opportunity to reconnect with yourself, reduce stress, and stay present.

Morning Rituals

How you begin your day influences the course of everything that comes after. Incorporating mindfulness into your morning routine can ground you and create a sense of calm before the day's demands take over.

- **Example:** Before checking your phone or diving into emails, take five minutes to focus on your breath or set an intention for the day.

    o *Prompt:* "What energy do I want to bring to today?"

    o *Technique:* Sit on the edge of your bed, close your eyes, and visualize your ideal day unfolding. This visualization creates a positive mindset.

- **Case Study: Nina's Calm Mornings** Nina, a school counselor, often started her mornings feeling rushed. She decided to dedicate ten minutes each morning to mindfulness journaling, jotting down three things she was grateful for and one intention for the day. This small change helped her feel more grounded and approach her work with a clear mind.

- **Interactive Exercise:** *Morning Mindfulness Plan*

    1. Identify one mindful practice to integrate into your morning (e.g., gratitude journaling, breathing exercises).

    2. Write down how you'll implement it for a week.

    3. Reflect on how this practice impacts your mood and focus throughout the day.

Mindfulness Cues Throughout the Day

Mindfulness doesn't have to be confined to a set time. Use everyday moments as reminders to pause and be present.

- **Examples of Mindfulness Cues:**

    o **Coffee Break:** While making or drinking coffee, focus on the aroma, taste, and warmth of the cup.

    o **Crossing Doorways:** Each time you walk through a doorway, take a deep breath and check in with how you're feeling.

o **Waiting Times:** Use moments in line or at red lights as opportunities to observe your breath or notice your surroundings.

- **Interactive Activity:** *Mindful Cue Tracker*

   1. Pick three cues to serve as mindfulness reminders (e.g., meal prep, brushing teeth, stepping outside).

   2. Track how often you remember to pause for mindfulness throughout the week.

   3. Reflect on any shifts in your awareness or mood.

Incorporating Technology Mindfully

Mindfulness and technology don't have to be at odds. Use apps and tools to enhance your practice rather than detract from it.

- **Examples of Mindful Technology Use:**

   o Download meditation apps like Calm or Headspace for guided sessions.

   o Set digital reminders to pause and breathe.

   o Use a timer to practice single-tasking during work hours.

- **Case Study: Sophia's Digital Mindfulness** Sophia, an online entrepreneur, felt constantly tethered to her devices. She began using an app that reminded her to take hourly mindfulness breaks. Over time, these pauses helped her feel more balanced and less reactive to constant notifications.

Overcoming Common Barriers

Despite the benefits of mindfulness, integrating it into daily life can be challenging. Addressing these barriers can help you stay consistent.

- **Common Challenges:**

  o *"I don't have time."* Start with micro-meditations or 1-2 minute practices.

  o *"It feels awkward or forced."* Focus on practices that resonate with you, like mindful eating or walking.

  o *"I forget to do it."* Use visual cues or alarms as reminders.

Interactive Exercise: Mindfulness Solutions Journal

1. Write down any barriers you face with mindfulness.

2. Brainstorm one or two practical solutions for each.

3. Test these strategies over a week and note improvements.

By weaving mindfulness into your daily routine, you create opportunities for calm and clarity amid life's busyness. Each small step builds a foundation for lasting change, helping you approach perfectionism and stress with balance and awareness. These practices are not about achieving a perfect state of mindfulness but about showing up for yourself in the present moment. As you integrate these strategies, you'll discover how mindfulness transforms the ordinary into something extraordinary, enriching your life with intention and presence.

Building Sustainable Habits and Long-Lasting Change

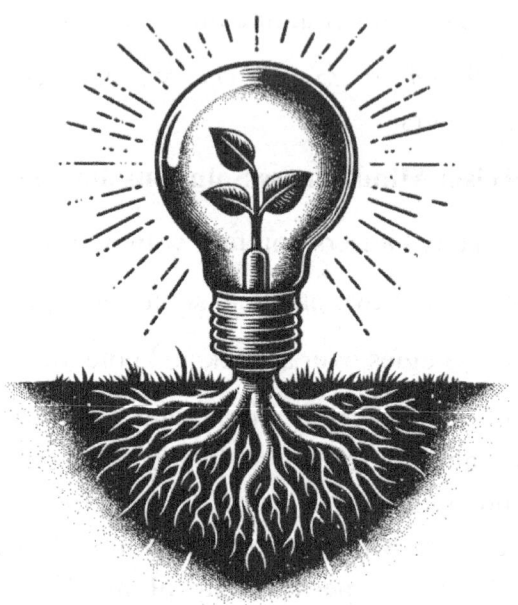

Picture this: waking up each morning with a sense of calm and clarity, your day unfolding with intention and ease. Imagine seamlessly transitioning from one task to another, each action aligned with your values and goals. It's not about perfection or control—it's about flow, a rhythm that carries you forward with purpose. This vision isn't some unattainable ideal; it's a tangible reality, made possible by the transformative power of habits.

Habits are the silent architects of our lives, weaving consistency into the fabric of our days. They shape routines, guide decisions, and influence behaviors that ultimately determine long-term success and fulfillment. From the moment you wake up to how you wind down at night, habits define how you navigate the world. But these habits don't have to form passively. By understanding the science of habit formation, you can take charge of this process, intentionally crafting routines that not only serve your goals but also bring balance and joy to your life.

At their core, habits free your mind from constant decision-making, creating space for creativity, focus, and emotional resilience. When thoughtfully cultivated, habits can help you break free from the constraints of perfectionism, replacing its rigid grip with flexibility and self-compassion. By leveraging the principles of habit formation, you can trade self-doubt for confidence, and overwhelm for clarity, creating a life where progress matters more than perfection.

Whether it's starting your morning with mindfulness, integrating small acts of gratitude throughout your day, or ending your evening with reflection, the habits you choose hold the power to rewrite your narrative. This chapter will guide you through understanding how habits work, the tools to build them intentionally, and strategies to sustain them. Together, we'll explore how small, consistent actions can lead to meaningful, lasting change, empowering you to design a life that aligns with your deepest values and aspirations.

9.1 Harnessing the Power of Habits

Habits act as the brain's autopilot system, allowing us to conserve mental energy for more complex and creative endeavors. At the heart of habit formation lies the habit loop, a simple yet powerful framework involving three components: **cue**, **routine**, and **reward**. This loop, popularized by Charles Duhigg in *The Power of Habit*, provides a roadmap for understanding how behaviors become automatic over time. The cue serves as the trigger that prompts the behavior, the routine is the action carried out, and the reward is the benefit that strengthens the likelihood of repeating the behavior.

Case Study: Ben's Writing Practice

Ben, an aspiring novelist, often found himself overwhelmed by the blank page. Despite his passion for storytelling, distractions like emails and social media often derailed his writing sessions. Determined to break the cycle, Ben designed a habit loop to transform his writing practice. His **cue** was brewing coffee each morning. Once his coffee was ready, he'd sit at his desk and write for 30 minutes— this became his **routine**. To make the habit enjoyable and sustainable, Ben **rewarded** himself with a short walk afterward, allowing him to reset his mind. Within a month, writing became an effortless daily habit, and Ben completed his novel draft ahead of schedule.

This example demonstrates how a thoughtfully designed habit loop can help you overcome obstacles and make meaningful progress toward your goals.

Strategies for Building Positive Habits

1. Start Small: Build Momentum with Manageable Goals

Overambitious goals can be daunting and lead to burnout. Starting small ensures that the habit feels achievable and sustainable. For example, begin with just 5 minutes of daily stretching rather than committing to a full workout right away. As the habit solidifies, you can gradually increase the intensity or duration. Small wins build confidence and create momentum, making it easier to maintain the habit over time.

Example: If you want to read more, commit to reading one page per day. Over time, you'll likely find yourself naturally reading more.

2. Tie Habits to Existing Routines

Known as habit stacking, this technique involves pairing a new habit with an established one. By anchoring the new behavior to an existing routine, you create a seamless transition that reduces the effort required to form the habit.

Example: To incorporate meditation, try linking it to your morning routine, like brushing your teeth. Once you've finished brushing, take a few moments to practice mindfulness. The established routine of brushing your teeth acts as the cue, reinforcing the new behavior.

Case Study: Beth's Water Intake Beth wanted to increase her daily water intake but often forgot. She decided to stack her habit onto her existing coffee routine. Each time she brewed a cup of coffee, she filled a glass of water and drank it before taking her first sip of coffee. This small adjustment helped her stay hydrated consistently.

3. Celebrate Wins: Reinforce the Behavior

Rewards play a crucial role in reinforcing habits, as they provide the brain with a sense of satisfaction. Immediate rewards are especially effective because they strengthen the association between the habit and the positive outcome.

Example: After completing a workout, treat yourself to a soothing playlist or a warm shower. These small acts of self-care help make the habit feel rewarding and enjoyable.

Tip: Use a rewards system that aligns with your values. For example, reward a week of consistent habits with something meaningful, like dedicating time to a favorite hobby.

Expanding Habit Awareness: Breaking Negative Cycles

While building positive habits is essential, breaking unhelpful ones is equally important. To disrupt negative cycles, identify the cues that trigger undesirable behaviors. Replace these cues with alternatives that support healthier habits.

Example: If you notice that stress triggers overeating, create a new habit loop:

- **Cue:** Feeling stressed after a meeting.
- **Routine:** Take a 5-minute walk instead of reaching for snacks.
- **Reward:** Enjoy a refreshing drink or spend a few moments stretching.

In time, replacing negative routines with positive ones helps you regain control and align your habits with your goals.

Habits are the building blocks of lasting change, operating quietly in the background to shape your life. By understanding and harnessing the power of the habit loop, you can transform your routines and behaviors, making progress feel natural and effortless. Start small, stack habits strategically, and celebrate every step forward. With time and consistency, you'll not only create habits that support your goals but also cultivate a life that reflects your aspirations and values.

9.2 Creating Long-Lasting Change Through Consistency

Consistency transforms fledgling habits into deeply ingrained routines. When habits are practiced regularly, neural pathways in the brain strengthen, making behaviors more automatic. This process, known as habit automation, is the key to sustaining long-term change.

Case Study: Priya's Fitness Routine

Priya wanted to exercise regularly but struggled with motivation. Instead of committing to hour-long sessions, she started with 10 minutes of yoga each morning. By staying consistent, Priya built confidence and gradually increased her workouts. Within six months, daily exercise became second nature.

Techniques to Maintain Consistency

1. **Habit Stacking**: Anchor new habits to existing ones. For example, journal for five minutes after pouring your morning coffee.

2. **Visual Reminders**: Place sticky notes, alarms, or habit trackers in visible locations to prompt action.

3. **Set Realistic Expectations**: Start small and increase gradually. Overcommitting often leads to burnout.

Overcoming Setbacks with Self-Compassion

No one is perfect, and setbacks are part of the process. Rather than giving up, reflect on what triggered the lapse and create a plan to avoid it in the future. Flexibility ensures that habits adapt to life's changes without being abandoned.

Interactive Activity: Consistency Tracker

- Create a weekly tracker with your target habits.

- Check off each day you complete the habit.

- At the end of the week, note your progress and celebrate small victories.

9.3 Personalized Action Plans for Sustained Success

A personalized action plan is your roadmap to meaningful change. By aligning your habits with your unique goals and values, you ensure that each step you take resonates deeply, fueling motivation and a sense of purpose. Crafting such a plan allows you to prioritize what truly matters, guiding you toward sustained success without burnout or overwhelm.

Anticipating Challenges and Adapting

No plan is foolproof, and challenges are inevitable. The key is to anticipate obstacles and develop contingency strategies.

Scenario Planning

Envision potential challenges and prepare responses:

- **Challenge:** Unexpected work demands.

- **Plan:** Adjust your goal (e.g., switch a 30-minute workout for a quick 10-minute stretch).

Case Study: Todd's Career Shift

Todd, a graphic designer transitioning to freelance work, faced inconsistent income and an unpredictable schedule. His action plan included:

1. Setting daily work hours for client projects.

2. Allocating time each week to pitch new clients.

3. Establishing an emergency fund for lean months.

By adapting his plan to address these challenges, Todd successfully transitioned to freelance work without compromising stability.

Reflection: Your Personalized Action Plan

Take a moment to reflect on your current goals and objectives. Use these prompts to guide your thinking:

1. What is one goal that aligns deeply with my values?

2. What small steps can I take to make this goal achievable?

3. How will I track my progress and adapt my plan as needed?

By crafting an action plan that reflects your unique priorities and leveraging tools to stay organized, you create a foundation for sustained success. Remember, progress is a journey, not a destination. Celebrate each step forward and allow your plan to evolve alongside your growth.

In the next section, we'll explore the importance of evaluating progress and adjusting strategies to ensure your goals remain dynamic and achievable. This iterative process will help you build resilience and adaptability, key components of long-term success.

9.4 Evaluating Progress and Adjusting Strategies

Evaluating progress is a critical step in maintaining momentum and refining strategies to achieve lasting success. Regular reflection helps you stay on track, recognize achievements, and identify areas where adjustments are needed. This process not only fosters a growth mindset but also ensures that your habits and plans evolve alongside your changing goals and circumstances.

Case Study: Ethan's Learning Journey

Ethan, a software developer, aimed to master a new programming language within six months. He initially relied on self-paced online courses but soon realized he was struggling to stay consistent. During his monthly progress review, Ethan identified his lack of accountability as a major obstacle. To address this, he joined a local study group of fellow developers. The group provided encouragement, shared resources, and offered a structure that helped Ethan stay committed. By the end of six months, not only had he mastered the basics of the language, but he also built meaningful connections with peers who supported his learning journey.

Key Components of Progress Evaluation

1. Set Key Performance Indicators (KPIs)

KPIs provide measurable benchmarks for tracking success. These indicators vary depending on your goals but should be specific and actionable.

Examples:

- For health goals: Track the number of daily steps or weekly exercise sessions.

- For professional development: Measure hours spent on skill-building or projects completed.

- For personal growth: Count days spent journaling or engaging in mindfulness practices.

Tip: Align KPIs with your SMART goals to ensure they are relevant and achievable.

Celebrate Milestones

Acknowledging achievements, no matter how small, boosts motivation and reinforces positive behaviors. Celebrating milestones creates a sense of accomplishment that propels you forward.

Ways to Celebrate:

- Treat yourself to something you enjoy, like a favorite meal or activity.

- Share your achievements with a friend or accountability partner.

- Reflect on how far you've come and what you've learned.

Interactive Exercise: Milestone Celebration Map

- List three milestones related to your goal.

- Write down specific ways you'll celebrate each milestone.

- Reflect on how these celebrations reinforce your commitment to your goals.

Overcoming Setbacks and Adjusting Strategies

Setbacks are inevitable, but they provide valuable opportunities for growth. By approaching them with self-compassion and curiosity, you can turn challenges into stepping stones for improvement.

1. Analyze Setbacks Without Judgment

When a setback occurs, resist the urge to criticize yourself. Instead, explore the factors that contributed to the lapse.

Example:

- **Setback:** Missing a week of workouts.

- **Analysis:** Long work hours and poor time management.

- **Adjustment:** Shift workouts to early mornings when energy levels are higher.

2. Embrace Flexibility

Rigid plans can falter in the face of unexpected changes. Flexibility allows you to adapt without abandoning your goals.

Case Study: Luke's Writing Schedule Luke, a freelance writer, planned to write for two hours every evening. When his schedule became unpredictable, he adjusted by writing for 30 minutes during lunch breaks. This small change allowed him to maintain consistency and progress.

3. Seek Feedback

Feedback from mentors, peers, or accountability partners offers fresh perspectives and constructive insights.

Exercise: Feedback Loop

- Identify someone you trust to review your progress.
- Ask for specific feedback on what's working and where improvements can be made.
- Use their input to refine your strategies.

Building a Feedback Loop for Continuous Improvement

A feedback loop ensures your goals and habits remain dynamic and responsive to your evolving needs.

Steps to Create a Feedback Loop:

1. **Set Regular Check-Ins:** Schedule biweekly or monthly reviews to assess progress.
2. **Reflect on Results:** Use tools like journals or progress trackers to identify patterns.

3. **Adjust as Needed:** Modify goals, timelines, or strategies based on what you've learned.

4. **Seek Support:** Share your progress with a mentor, coach, or peer for additional insights.

Example: If your goal is to save money, a feedback loop might include reviewing your budget monthly, analyzing spending trends, and adjusting savings targets based on unexpected expenses.

Final Reflection: Tracking and Adjusting for Success

Reflect on these questions to enhance your progress evaluation process:

- What methods am I using to track my progress, and are they effective?

- How do I celebrate milestones to stay motivated?

- What adjustments can I make to ensure my strategies remain relevant and achievable?

By regularly evaluating your progress and adapting your approach, you build resilience and flexibility, ensuring your habits continue to serve you. Remember, progress is a journey filled with learning and growth, and every step forward brings you closer to your goals.

In our final chapter, we'll explore the power of a growth mindset and how it can transform your relationship with challenges, enabling you to thrive in an ever-changing world.

Cultivating A Growth Mindset

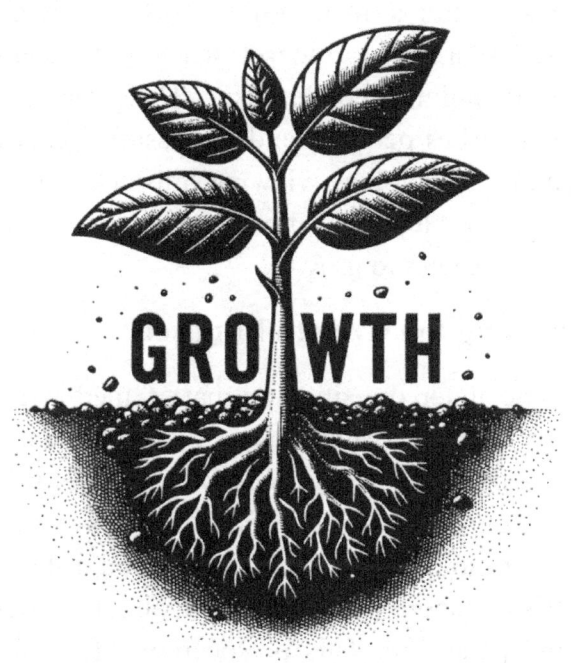

Imagine a young child learning to ride a bicycle. Each wobble, fall, and scraped knee is met with determination rather than defeat. This child embodies a growth mindset, viewing each attempt as a steppingstone toward mastery. Contrast this with a child who gives up after one fall, convinced they lack the talent to succeed. This illustrates a fixed mindset, where abilities and intelligence are seen as static, unchangeable traits. Psychologist Carol Dweck's groundbreaking research on growth mindsets underscores the principle that intelligence, skills, and capabilities are not fixed but can be developed through effort, resilience, and learning. For anyone striving to manage perfectionism, this mindset offers a powerful tool for embracing challenges, persisting through obstacles, and celebrating progress over perfection.

A growth mindset reframes challenges as opportunities for development rather than threats to self-worth. It encourages resilience, curiosity, and a focus on the process over immediate results. In contrast, a fixed mindset leads individuals to avoid challenges, fearing failure and criticism. This fear creates a self-limiting cycle that stifles personal and professional growth. Shifting to a growth mindset involves viewing mistakes as natural and valuable parts of the learning process, fostering a passion for discovery and an openness to growth.

10.1 Understanding the Growth Mindset

Have you ever encountered a situation that seemed insurmountable, only to look back later and realize it was a turning point for growth? This shift often depends on your mindset. A growth mindset, a term coined by psychologist Carol Dweck, reflects the belief that intelligence and abilities can be cultivated through hard work and perseverance. It's not about innate talent but about the willingness to learn, adapt, and persevere. This perspective differs from a fixed mindset, which assumes that abilities and intelligence are unalterable traits. Understanding the difference between these perspectives is the foundation for personal and professional transformation.

When we operate with a growth mindset, we approach challenges as opportunities rather than threats. We become curious instead of fearful, persistent instead of defeated. This mindset fuels resilience, creativity, and innovation, enabling us to thrive in dynamic environments. Shifting from a fixed mindset to a growth-oriented perspective is not always easy, especially in the face of setbacks or deeply ingrained beliefs. However, with intentionality and practice, it is possible to rewire how we think about ourselves and our abilities.

Case Study: Craig's Professional Pivot

Craig, a seasoned marketing executive, encountered a significant challenge when his company adopted a complex new software platform. He initially resisted the change, convinced he "wasn't tech-savvy enough" to master it. His fixed mindset made him feel inadequate, frustrated, and overwhelmed.

One day, a colleague introduced him to the principles of a growth mindset, encouraging him to view the situation as an opportunity to expand his skill set. Craig started reframing his thoughts. Instead of saying, "I can't do this," he began telling himself, "I can learn this step by step." He sought training sessions, allocated daily practice time, and celebrated small milestones, such as successfully navigating a tricky feature.

Over a few months, Craig not only became proficient with the platform but also uncovered innovative ways to leverage its tools for his team. His newfound confidence and skills earned him a leadership opportunity in a company-wide project. What began as a daunting challenge turned into a career milestone, all because of his decision to embrace growth over resistance.

The Neuroscience of Growth

The power of the growth mindset is rooted in the brain's incredible adaptability, known as neuroplasticity. Our brains form new connections when we engage in learning and practice, reinforcing pathways that support new skills and habits. This means that with effort and persistence, it's possible to develop abilities that once seemed beyond reach. For Craig, this meant rewiring his brain to view technical skills as learnable rather than out of his grasp.

Neuroplasticity underscores the importance of consistent effort and intentional practice. The more we approach challenges with curiosity and determination, the more we strengthen neural pathways that support resilience and adaptability. This biological foundation offers

184

hope and a roadmap for anyone looking to shift from a fixed to a growth mindset.

Takeaway

Understanding and adopting a growth mindset isn't an overnight transformation—it's a practice. By recognizing when you're operating with a fixed mindset and choosing to reframe challenges as opportunities, you unlock the potential for continuous learning and development. Like Craig, you can turn obstacles into achievements and create a foundation for long-term growth.

10.2 Shifting from Fixed to Growth Mindset

Consider standing at the edge of a challenging new opportunity—whether it's starting a project, learning a skill, or navigating a life change. Your initial thoughts might set the tone for your journey. Do you hear an inner voice saying, "I'm not cut out for this," or, "This is my chance to grow"? This inner dialogue reflects the difference between a fixed mindset and a growth mindset. Transitioning to a growth mindset begins with awareness of these thought patterns and a commitment to transforming them into tools for resilience and optimism.

The Power of Reframing

A growth mindset thrives on reframing. Rather than viewing failure as evidence of inadequacy, it reframes it as an opportunity for growth and for improvement. Reframing is not just a mental trick—it's a practice of looking at situations through a lens of opportunity rather than limitation.

Example: Overcoming Setbacks

Suppose you applied for a promotion but didn't get the position. A fixed mindset might say, "I'll never be good enough for that role." A growth mindset, however, reframes the experience: "This gives me insight into what I need to work on. I'll use the feedback to grow and try again." By adopting this perspective, setbacks become a source of motivation rather than a roadblock.

Interactive Activity: Reframe and Rethink

Write down a recent setback or challenge. Then, create two columns:

- **Fixed Mindset Response:** Write how you initially felt or reacted.

- **Growth Mindset Reframe:** Reframe the situation as an opportunity for learning or growth.

Case Study: Michelle's Return to School

Michelle, a mother of two, decided to return to college after years away from academics. The first semester was overwhelming, and she found herself questioning her decision: "Am I too old for this? Can I keep up?"

One of her professors introduced her to the concept of a growth mindset. Michelle began to focus on steady effort, setting small, achievable goals for herself each week. She also sought support from peers and professors, recognizing that asking for help was part of the process.

By shifting her perspective and celebrating incremental progress, Michelle found her confidence growing. Over time, she not only adapted but excelled, graduating with honors. Her success stemmed from her ability to reframe challenges as opportunities to learn and grow.

Building Momentum

Shifting to a growth mindset is a gradual process, requiring intention and practice. By reframing failures, cultivating self-awareness, and seeking feedback, you begin to see yourself not as a fixed entity but as a work in progress. Each step forward, no matter how small, reinforces this shift, creating momentum that empowers you to tackle new challenges with confidence and curiosity.

10.3 Lifelong Learning as a Foundation for Growth

Imagine the excitement of discovering something new—a skill, a perspective, or a piece of knowledge that changes how you see the world. Lifelong learning is about embracing that sense of wonder and curiosity, ensuring that growth becomes a natural and ongoing part of your life. It's not just about formal education; it's about seizing opportunities to learn from experiences, people, and the ever-changing world around you. A commitment to lifelong learning keeps your mind agile, your perspective fresh, and your potential limitless.

The Power of Lifelong Learning

Lifelong learners thrive because they view knowledge not as a finite resource but as an endless journey. This mindset fuels adaptability, resilience, and innovation. Studies show that continuous learning improves mental health, boosts problem-solving skills, and fosters a sense of purpose. Whether learning a new language, delving into a creative hobby, or mastering a professional skill, the benefits extend far beyond the practical—lifelong learning enriches your life and keeps you connected to the world around you.

Case Study: James's Career Renaissance

James, a mid-level manager, found himself feeling stagnant in his career. Rather than settle, he decided to enroll in a data analytics course—a field he'd always been curious about but had no prior experience in. The course was challenging, but James embraced the process, asking for help when needed and applying his learning to his current role. His new skills not only reinvigorated his passion for work but also opened doors to leadership opportunities. James's commitment to lifelong learning transformed his career trajectory and reignited his enthusiasm for growth.

Exploring Different Modes of Learning

Lifelong learning isn't limited to traditional methods. Embrace a variety of approaches to keep your journey dynamic and engaging.

Examples:

- **Online Courses:** Platforms like Coursera or Udemy offer accessible ways to dive into new topics.

- **Podcasts and Audiobooks:** Great for learning on the go, these formats are perfect for busy schedules.

- **Workshops and Conferences:** In-person events provide hands-on learning and networking opportunities.

- **Hobbies:** Activities like painting, gardening, or playing an instrument can unlock creativity and mindfulness while building new skills.

Case Study: Jessica's Creative Outlet

Jessica, a busy entrepreneur, felt burned out by the demands of her business. She decided to take a pottery class as a way to explore something unrelated to her work. The process of creating with her hands was both therapeutic and inspiring, reigniting her creativity. She soon found that the lessons she learned in pottery—like patience and embracing imperfection—translated to her professional life as well.

Celebrating the Journey

Lifelong learning is as much about the process as it is about the outcomes. Celebrate your progress, no matter how small, and recognize the effort you've put into expanding your horizons. Whether it's mastering a new skill or gaining a fresh perspective, each step is a testament to your commitment to growth.

By embracing lifelong learning, you cultivate a mindset that values curiosity, resilience, and the joy of discovery. This approach not only enhances your personal and professional life but also prepares you to navigate the ever-changing world with confidence and adaptability.

10.4 Embracing Self-Discovery

Self-discovery is not a destination but a lifelong journey—a continuous unfolding of your true self through experiences, reflection, and growth. It is about peeling back layers of external expectations and connecting with the values, strengths, and passions that make you uniquely you. This process empowers you to live authentically, make aligned decisions, and navigate life with a sense of purpose. By embracing self-discovery, you create a foundation for personal and professional growth, resilience, and fulfillment.

Tools for Self-Discovery

1. **Values Inventory**
   Your values act as the guiding compass for your choices and actions. Identifying your core values helps you prioritize what truly matters and align your actions accordingly.

How to Create a Values Inventory:

   o Write down 20 values that resonate with you (e.g., honesty, creativity, family, freedom).

   o Refine the list to highlight your five most essential core values.

   o Reflect on how these values influence your daily life and long-term goals.

Example:

Kristina discovered that "creativity" and "connection" were her top values. She realized her job as an accountant felt unfulfilling because it didn't align with these values. This clarity motivated her to transition into a creative role in marketing, where she now thrives.

Community Connection

Surrounding yourself with supportive and inspiring individuals creates an environment that nurtures self-discovery. These relationships provide perspective, encouragement, and accountability as you explore your potential.

Interactive Activity: Build Your Growth Circle

- Identify three people who inspire or uplift you.

- Reach out to each person and schedule a conversation to share goals, challenges, and reflections.

- Regularly meet to support one another's journeys of self-discovery.

Case Study: Noah's Path to Authenticity

Noah, a successful attorney, often felt disconnected from his work. After taking a values inventory, he realized his top values—freedom, creativity, and adventure—were missing from his career. Through mindfulness and journaling, Noah connected with his childhood passion for storytelling. Encouraged by his growth circle, he started writing in his free time, eventually publishing his first novel. While he continues practicing law, Noah now feels fulfilled by balancing his career with his passion.

Interactive Assessment: The Self-Discovery Map

This final activity is designed to create a tangible representation of your self-discovery journey, offering clarity and direction for the future.

Step 1: Reflection

- Identify key moments in your life where you felt most authentic and fulfilled.

- Write down the skills, values, and passions that emerged during these moments.

Step 2: Mapping Your Strengths

- Draw a circle in the center of a blank page. Write "ME" inside it.

- Around the circle, list your top five strengths, values, and passions.

Step 3: Setting Your North Star

- At the top of the page, write your "North Star"—a short statement that encapsulates your purpose or ultimate goal. *Example: "Fostering meaningful connections through the art of storytelling."*

Step 4: Planning Your Path

- Draw arrows connecting your central circle to your North Star.

- On each arrow, write specific actions or goals that will help you align with your North Star.

Step 5: Reflect and Commit

- Review your map and identify one small step you can take today toward living authentically.

Celebrating the Journey

Self-discovery is not about finding a final answer but about embracing the process of learning, evolving, and growing. Celebrate your progress by recognizing how far you've come, no matter where you are in your journey.

Gratitude Reflection:

Write a letter to your past self, acknowledging the courage and growth that have brought you to this point. Share your hopes and encouragement for the next stage of your journey.

By embracing self-discovery, you unlock the potential to lead a life that resonates with your deepest aspirations. This chapter—and the entire workbook—are the building blocks toward a more authentic and fulfilling life. Keep in mind: You are your most important project, and every step forward is a triumph to be celebrated.

Conclusion: A Journey Toward Growth and Fulfillment

As you arrive at the end of this workbook, take a moment to honor the journey you've embarked upon and the progress you've made. Together, we've navigated the intricate layers of perfectionism, not to erase it, but to transform it into a catalyst for growth, self-discovery, and fulfillment.

Through these chapters, you've explored powerful tools to confront and reframe perfectionism—tools rooted in self-compassion, emotional resilience, and intentional living. We've delved into the nuances of embracing imperfection, fostering mindfulness, overcoming procrastination, and building habits that align with your values. From learning to delegate with trust to adopting a growth mindset, each strategy has been a step forward in reclaiming your time and energy for what truly matters.

This journey has been about more than strategies; it's been about empowerment. The insights and practices shared here are designed to help you build a foundation for lasting change. They are an invitation to cultivate self-awareness, treat yourself with kindness, and approach life with resilience and adaptability. By adopting a growth mindset, you've opened yourself to a world of continuous learning and possibility. These are not just tools—they are a way of life, one that honors your unique strengths and aspirations.

A Message of Hope and Encouragement

Know that change is within your reach. Each small step you take, no matter how modest, has the potential to spark profound transformation. Begin with one or two strategies that resonate most with you, integrating them into your daily life with intention. Allow yourself the grace to move at your own pace, knowing that progress is not linear but deeply personal.

Challenges will arise, as they do for all of us. When they do, remember that they are not roadblocks but opportunities to grow stronger and wiser. Each setback is a chance to reflect, recalibrate, and press forward with even greater clarity. Keep a journal of your journey—celebrate the victories, learn from the missteps, and watch how far you've come. This practice will serve as a testament to your resilience and commitment to becoming the best version of yourself.

Gratitude and Connection

As we conclude, I want to express my heartfelt gratitude to you for engaging with this workbook. It has been a privilege to share these insights and strategies with you, drawn from my own journey and research. Knowing that these pages have the potential to make a difference in your life fills me with hope and purpose.

This is not a goodbye but an invitation to stay connected. You are not alone on this path. Explore the companion resources available to support your continued growth and consider joining online communities where you can share your experiences and learn from others. Together, we can create a network of encouragement and inspiration that fosters lasting change.

Your Next Chapter

This workbook is a tool, but the true transformation lies in how you apply what you've learned. Revisit these pages as often as you need, using them as a guidepost in moments of doubt or renewal. Trust in your ability to manage perfectionism's hold and live a life aligned with your values and aspirations. You are capable of so much more than you realize, and every step forward is a testament to your strength and courage.

Thank you for giving me the opportunity to join you on this journey. As you step into the next chapter of your life, do so with confidence, self-compassion, and the unshakable belief that you have the power to create a life of meaning and joy. One step at a time, you are transforming not just how you live—but how you thrive.

References

Adler, A. (n.d.). Alfred Adler's personality theory and personality types. *Journal Psyche*. https://journalpsyche.org/alfred-adler-personality-theory/

Asana. (n.d.). The Eisenhower matrix: How to prioritize your to-do list. https://asana.com/resources/eisenhower-matrix

Business Insider. (n.d.). 29 famous people who failed before they succeeded. https://www.businessinsider.com/successful-people-who-failed-at-first-2015-7

Choosing Therapy. (n.d.). How to overcome your inner critic. https://www.choosingtherapy.com/overcome-inner-critic/

Clear, J. (n.d.). How to build new habits by taking advantage of old ones. https://jamesclear.com/habit-stacking

Clear, J. (n.d.). Keystone habits: The simple way to improve all aspects of your life. https://jamesclear.com/keystone-habits

Cornell University Graduate School.(n.d.) Changing your fixed mindset into a growth mindset.https://gradschool.cornell.edu/alumni/alumni-newsletter-spring-2019/changing-your-fixed-mindset-into-a-growth-mindset/

Culture Partners. (n.d.). Mastering psychological flexibility: Building resilience. https://culturepartners.com/insights/mastering-psychological-flexibility-building-resilience/

Dweck, C. S. (2006). *Mindset: The new psychology of success.* Random House.

Fast Company. (n.d.). 10-time management apps that CEOs swear by. https://www.fastcompany.com/91140850/10-time-management-apps-that-ceos-swear-by Flourish Psychology. (n.d.). How to use CBT to manage fear.

https://flourishpsychologynyc.com/how-to-use-cbt-to-manage-fear/

Georgetown University Medical Center. (2023, November 9). Mindfulness-based stress reduction is as effective as an antidepressant drug for treating anxiety disorders. https://gumc.georgetown.edu/news-release/mindfulness-based-stress-reduction-is-as-effective-as-an-antidepressant-drug-for-treating-anxiety-disorders/

Happily.ai. (n.d.). Personal SWOT analysis: A comprehensive guide for personal development. https://blog.happily.ai/personal-swot-analysis-a-comprehensive-guide-for-personal-development/

Harvard Business Review. (2024, January). How high-performing teams build trust. https://hbr.org/2024/01/how-high-performing-teams-build-trust

Harvard Business School Online. (n.d.). How to delegate effectively: 9 tips for managers. https://online.hbs.edu/blog/post/how-to-delegate-effectively

Healthline. (n.d.). Cognitive restructuring: Techniques and examples. https://www.healthline.com/health/cognitive-restructuring

Healthline. (n.d.). The science of habit: How to rewire your brain. https://www.healthline.com/health/the-science-of-habit

Indeed. (n.d.). How to write SMART goals in 5 steps (with examples). https://www.indeed.com/career-advice/career-development/how-to-write-smart-goals

Mayo Clinic. (n.d.). Mindfulness exercises.
https://www.mayoclinic.org/healthy-lifestyle/consumer-
health/in-depth/mindfulness-exercises/art-20046356

Mayo Clinic. (n.d.). Resilience: Build skills to endure hardship.
https://www.mayoclinic.org/tests-procedures/resilience-
training/in-depth/resilience/art-20046311

Medical News Today. (n.d.). Controlling people: Signs, causes, and
how to deal with them.
https://www.medicalnewstoday.com/articles/controlling-
people

Medium. (n.d.). Procrastination CBT techniques to overcome
procrastination. https://medium.com/syndicate-
post/procrastination-cbt-techniques-to-overcome-
procrastination-a9781b0e0c1a

Mindset Works. (n.d.). The growth mindset - What is growth
mindset? https://www.mindsetworks.com/science/

Motion. (n.d.). Single-tasking: Mastering the art of deep, productive
work. https://www.usemotion.com/blog/single-tasking

Neff, K. (n.d.). Self-compassion research by Kristin Neff. Self-
Compassion website: https://self-compassion.org/the-
research/

PubMed Central. (n.d.). Focus on self-presentation on social media
is associated...
https://pmc.ncbi.nlm.nih.gov/articles/PMC11389274/

PubMed Central. (n.d.). Multidimensional models of perfectionism
and procrastination.
https://pmc.ncbi.nlm.nih.gov/articles/PMC7400384/

PubMed Central. (n.d.). Neural plasticity of development and
    learning.
    https://pmc.ncbi.nlm.nih.gov/articles/PMC6871182/

Positive Psychology. (n.d.). What is mindful self-compassion?

(Incl exercises + PDF).https://positivepsychology.com/mindful-self-
    compassion/

Psych Central. (2015). Understanding the root cause of
    perfectionism.
    https://psychcentral.com/blog/imperfect/2015/12/what-
    causes-perfectionism

Psych Central. (n.d.). Mindfulness & gratitude: Why and how they
    should pair.https://psychcentral.com/blog/how-gratitude-and-
    mindfulness-go-hand-in-hand

Psychology Today. (n.d.). How to defend your boundaries and be
    assertive.https://www.psychologytoday.com/us/blog/the-
    wisdom-of-anger/202312/how-to-defend-your-boundaries-
    and-be-assertive

SAP. (n.d.). Addressing digital distractions to focus on
    work.https://www.sap.com/france/insights/viewpoints/addres
    sing-digital-distractions.html

SessionLab. (n.d.). 14 effective feedback techniques and methods
    for giving
    feedback.https://www.sessionlab.com/blog/feedback-
    techniques/

Shawnee-KS. (n.d.). The curse of perfectionism: Why it hinders
    workplace productivity.https://www.shawnee-
    ks.com/2024/02/27/the-curse-of-perfectionism-why-it-
    hinders-workplace-productivity/

Tactyqal. (n.d.) 25 entrepreneurs who failed before becoming successful.https://www.tactyqal.com/blog/25-entrepreneurs-who-failed-before-becoming-successful/

The New Hope Mental Health Counseling Services. (n.d.). The power of acceptance: Embracing imperfection in your partner.https://www.thenewhopemhcs.com/the-power-of-acceptance-embracing-imperfection-in-your-partner/

Todoist. (n.d.). Paralyzed by perfectionism? Try rethinking your to-do list.https://todoist.com/inspiration/dealing-with-perfectionism-todo-list

Wegerer, M. (2024). Cognitive-behavioral treatment of perfectionism. https://doi.org/10.1159/000532044

https://karger.com/ver/article/34/1/1/862136/Cognitive-Behavioral-Treatment-of-Perfectionism-An

About the Author

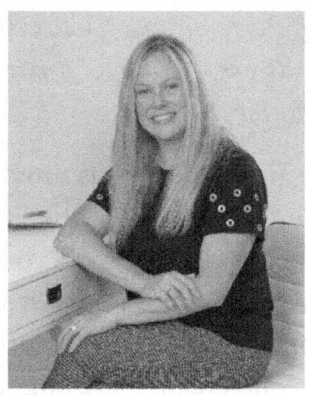

Stacey Bottone, Ed.D., combines nearly two decades of experience in education with a deep commitment to personal growth and development. A graduate of Nebraska Methodist College, Dr. Bottone has dedicated her career to empowering others to manage the barriers that hinder progress.

Drawing from her own experiences and extensive research, Stacey's approach is both compassionate and relatable, offering readers insights that inspire real change. Her Detox Workbook series reflects her belief in progress over perfection and her commitment to helping others achieve their goals without compromising their well-being.

Dr. Bottone resides in northeastern Connecticut with her husband, Josh, and their three beloved Labrador rescues. Her son and daughter-in-law live in Central Pennsylvania. A lifelong learner and advocate for holistic self-improvement, Stacey is dedicated to creating resources that empower readers to thrive in both their personal and professional lives.

For more information visit: www.staceybottone.com

Thank You for Reading!

Thank you for reading *Perfectionist Detox Workbook: 9 Practical Strategies to Alleviate Stress, Manage Anxiety, and Reclaim Your Time for What Really Matters!*

I hope *Perfectionist Detox Workbook* has provided you with valuable insights and actionable strategies to alleviate perfectionism and reclaim a sense of balance and purpose in your life. Whether you're striving for personal growth, building resilience, or seeking to live more authentically, I hope this guide has empowered you to embrace progress over perfection and create a life aligned with your values.

If you found this book helpful (or even if you just have a moment to share your thoughts), I would be incredibly grateful if you could leave a review on Amazon. As an independent author, your feedback helps me reach more readers and continue creating resources that inspire growth and transformation. Every review, no matter how brief, truly makes a difference.

Thank you so much for your support!

Warmly,

Stacey Bottone

Made in the USA
Monee, IL
17 March 2025

14109380R00115